THE SELF-HEALING BLUEPRINT: LEARN HOW TO BECOME YOUR OWN HEALTH EXPERT

From Patient to Provider

ANTHONY MARTINEZ BEVEN

NPI Registered Nutritional Detox Specialist, Naturopathic Practitioner, Homeopath, & Health Educator

© Anthony Martinez Beven | Become Publishing

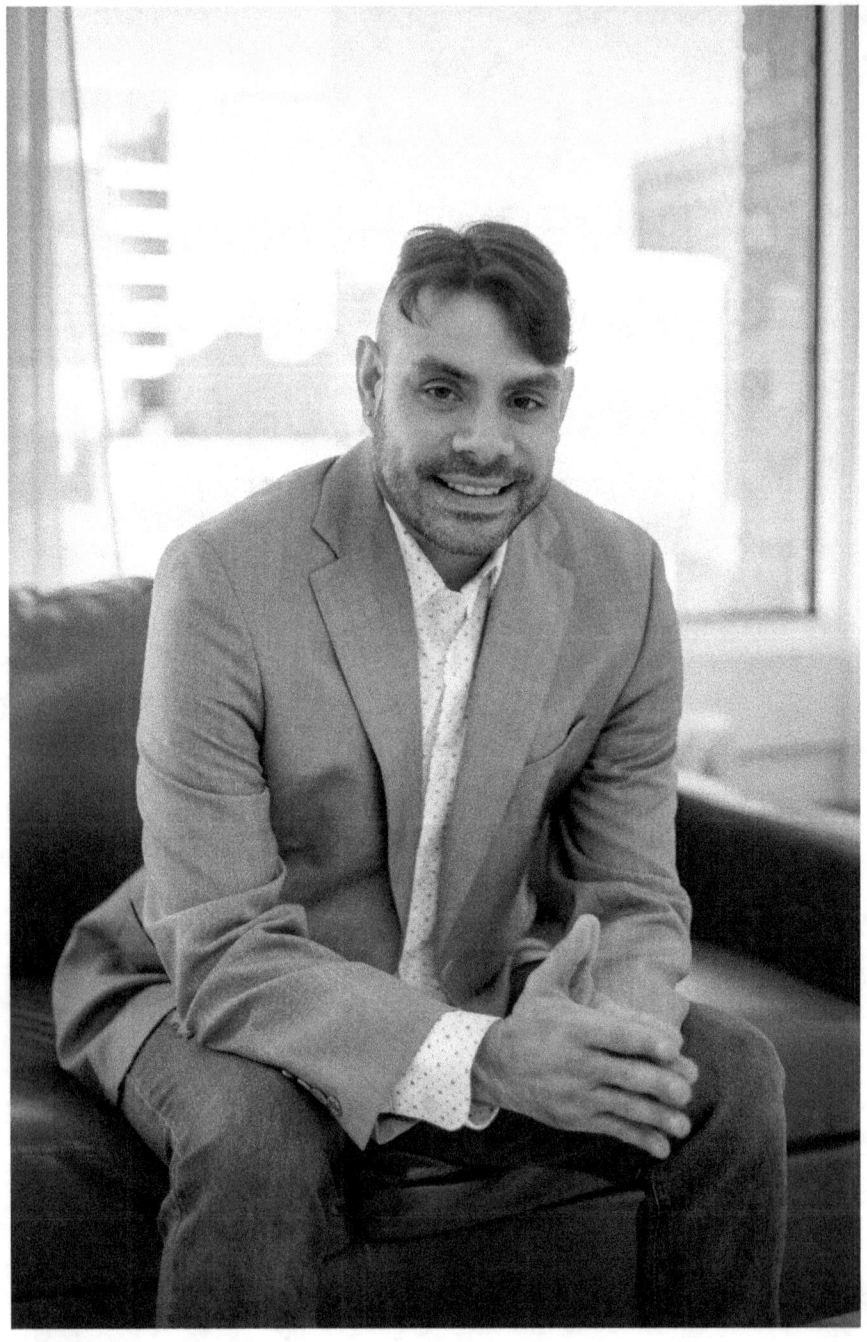

PREFACE

I dedicate this book to my grandparents, Carmen and Trinidad Martinez. Gram, you showed me love, kindness, and compassion. Grandpa, you taught me integrity, honesty, and detox. I miss you, and I love you both.

Thank you for purchasing this book. I'd like to begin with what I've learned over the years and how you can apply my experiences, knowledge, and lessons in your own healing journey.

There is a systematic attack on the human body from a global corporate conglomerate structure to keep you in a sick care system that doesn't address illness at its root cause.

That's what I discovered in my situation.

I'm mutated on five of six methylation genes, one of the key gene groups responsible for core cellular-level conversions and breakdowns. My body doesn't properly break down a key amino acid found in meat protein due to MTHFR genetic mutations. I also can't convert folate to usable form, or properly metabolize the male forms of estrogen for hormonal balance. One of the main functions of hormones is cellular-level communication.

Most of my inflammation response genes are mutated,

and I'm missing the gene that codes for stage 2 of the liver detox process: blood cleansing for pre-carcinogens and environmental toxins.

This was the underlying cause of my HIV and cancer back-to-back diagnoses in 2017; bouts with ocular herpes, shingles, kidney stones and COVID; and another undiagnosed fight with cancer, and subsequent shingles, and COVID again in late 2022 through much of 2023.

My story isn't unique.

Approximately 60% of Americans are living with one or more chronic illnesses, according to the Centers for Disease Control. The top causes of death in America are 1) heart disease, 2) cancer, and 3) misdiagnosis. Medical doctors can't properly diagnose patients because they don't know enough about biochemical processes, cellular-level functionality, and DNA/genetics.

The pharmaceutical industry, which is part of the corporate conglomerate system, sits on the curriculum boards of all the major medical schools in America.

Doctors are also governed by medical boards, which uphold scientific research as "evidence-based." However, scientific integrity has been called into question.

The Dana-Farber Cancer Institute, a Harvard Medical School affiliate, announced in January 2024 that it's requesting retractions and corrections of 37 scientific papers due to "data forgery." The investigation was launched by a blogger and reported by multiple news outlets, including the student newspaper, The Harvard Crimson.

Doctors are trained to on medications, medical procedures,

surgeries, and vaccinations. Most doctors have little to no training in utilizing food as medicine or alternative healing therapies.

Patients are often misdiagnosed several times before receiving a proper diagnosis, if they ever do. They are put on the wrong medications or the wrong combination of medications. They undergo the wrong medical procedures or surgeries, resulting in death or some form of serious harm that causes a disability.

We live and operate within a system built on limiting beliefs. One of those beliefs is your "doctor knows best." Sick patients are the profit centers in this system.

You are conditioned to believe that doctors are in control of your health. You are in control of your health and only you.

Now, it's time to become your own health expert.

TABLE OF CONTENTS

INTRODUCTION
CHAPTER 1: EXPOSURE TO TOXINS
CHAPTER 2: THE DIAGNOSIS
CHAPTER 3: THE POWER
CHAPTER 4: THE ART & SCIENCE OF DETOX
CHAPTER 5: YOUR BODY, YOUR MACHINE
CHAPTER 6: DETOX DAY SPA
CHAPTER 7: DNA & KEY GENE GROUPS
CHAPTER 8: THE DIGESTIVE SYSTEM & ACCESSORY ORGANS
CHAPTER 9: CELL DEBRIS & FREE RADICALS
CHAPTER 10: HEAVY METAL TOXICITY
CHAPTER 11: PAIN & INFLAMMATION
CHAPTER 12: MOLD TOXICITY & DETOX
CHAPTER 13: BLOOD CLEANSING & REBUILD
CHAPTER 14: HORMONAL IMBALANCE
CHAPTER 15: ANXIETY & THE MAGNESIUM FIX
CHAPTER 16: CANCER A.K.A. SEVERE OXIDATIVE STRESS
CHAPTER 17: THE GUT-BRAIN AXIS
CHAPTER 18: DERMAL DETOX
CHAPTER 19: WEIGHT LOSS & WEIGHT GAIN
CHAPTER 20: HAIR LOSS & TOOTH LOSS
CHAPTER 21: GENETIC TESTING & DETOXING FOR CHILDREN
CHAPTER 22: MTHFR & PREGNANT MOMS
CHAPTER 23: CELLULAR FUNCTIONALITY & THE CELL CYCLE
CHAPTER 24: NUTRIENT DEFICIENT FOOD &

SUPPLEMENTS
CHAPTER 25: SUPER SUPPLEMENTS, COMBINATIONS & RX INTERACTIONS
CHAPTER 26: FOOD CONSUMPTION
CHAPTER 27: PROPER HYDRATION
CHAPTER 28: EYE DISEASE, DETOX & IRIDOLOGY
CHAPTER 29: LUNG DETOX
CHAPTER 30: FASTING
CHAPTER 31: SELF-ASSESSMENT & MEDICAL TESTING
CHAPTER 32: BECOME YOUR OWN HEALTH EXPERT

INTRODUCTION

> Disclaimer: Althought I'm a wellness practitioner, I would like to clarify that I am not a medical doctor. My services are based on holistic approaches and alternative therapies, which may complement conventional medical treatments but should not be considered a substitute for professional medical advice, diagnosis, or treatment. It is important to consult with a qualified healthcare provider for any medical concerns or conditions.

My journey started around 10 months old when I received the Pertussis vaccine. I experienced a severe reaction, and my veins weren't large enough for an IV to address the situation. An incision had to be made in the back of my head instead.

My body's impaired immune function couldn't defend against and detox the vaccine's toxic additives, including aluminum phosphate, formaldehyde, glutaraldehyde, and 2-phenoxyethanol.

I experienced gastrointestinal issues throughout my 20s and 30s, and in 2017, at 34, I received back-to-back in HIV and cancer. I was faced with a life-and-death crisis.

My genetic testing revealed that my body would be receptive to five of the approximately 30 HIV medications available at the time, and the first medication my doctor prescribed was denied by insurance.

I was getting sicker, and the only medical solution during this waiting game was to load my system with vaccines and possibly chemo pills.

Once again, my whole body was in inflammation, and I needed resolution fast. But, something inside of me — my higher self, said, "No, this won't work."

I communicated that to my doctor, who asked what I wanted to do.

I instinctively replied, "Flush my body, reset and reboot my immune system."

So, that's what I did.

All the nutritionists and naturopaths I spoke to didn't have the knowledge or clinical experience to address what was happening to me. I didn't know what was happening to me, but I knew they couldn't help me. I had to do it myself.

I figured out how to manifest the self-healing I needed. I took the power back from my doctors to become my own health expert.

In 2022, I battled COVID twice. In early 2023, I was up against back-to-back bouts with shingles, another undiagnosed second bout with cancer, and an asthma resurgence from childhood that left my body depleted of energy and mineral content.

I could barely get out of bed, and even walking a few hundred feet winded me. This time, I tapped into my subconscious mind to access knowledge of ancient healing methods and how to remove trauma blocks impacting my physical body.

I've gone through it to help you get through it with confidence, a stronger sense of self, and real-world applications for self-healing through a concrete understanding of human anatomy/biology, cellular level functionality, DNA/genetics, nutritional science, and more.

Let's embrace this journey to the center of the universe, all within you. In these pages, I will address what I've learned in becoming my own health expert:

1. No one is going to love, care for, or support you more than you.
2. Trust yourself. You are always right. Whether you are or not, you're going to do what you want to do. You'll learn your lessons and maybe other important ones along the way to figuring it out.
3. Your health is 100% your responsibility: no one else's — not your doctor's, not your therapist's, no one but YOURS.
4. Our bodies are machines. They either break down or convert, but our machines are malfunctioning or busted.
5. The underlying genetic cause of all chronic, physical illnesses is mutations or deletions within the human genetic code, which codes the body to these breakdowns and conversions.
6. Our air, food, water, personal-care products, cookware, medications, and medical testing contain heavy metals and other toxic, pre-carcinogenic ingredients.
7. Everyone has mitochondrial disease. The mitochondria are the brain, the powerhouse of the cell, responsible for energy input and output, cell

protection and more.
8. Our gut is our second brain, and our gut microbiome is compromised resulting in leaky gut, which causes the blood to become low-to-mid grade septic.
9. Enzymes with mineral cofactors are required to start all the biochemical processes inside the body. No one has enzyme functionality because the accessory organs (liver, gallbladder, and pancreas) are inflamed from food, water, and medications that contain toxic additives and are nutrient-deficient and mineral deficient.
10. Our bodies are mineral deficient, particularly for the main two minerals required for enzyme processes — magnesium and zinc — which play a role in 300 enzyme processes separately. Iron, calcium, and potassium round out the top five remaining minerals that act as enzymatic cofactors.
11. The food is nutrient and mineral-deficient and, in many cases, genetically modified.
12. Our bodies are full of toxic heavy metals, such as gadolinium, mercury, and aluminum, and lack positive metals, such as copper and zinc, that the body needs.
13. Every decade you are sick requires one full year of consistent and comprehensive internal and external detox activities.
14. Women are not metabolizing and breaking down estrogen — and men aren't either for the male form of estrogen — due to genetic mutations with their COMT gene in the methylation group.
15. Most people aren't effectively metabolizing proteins — either plant or meat. This is due to mutations with MTHFR allele C677T, which is responsible for breaking down amino acid

homocysteine to methionine. This amino acid is the key building block for protein. Too many undigested proteins convert to fats and sugars.

16. Most people aren't effectively converting folate, which is mainly found in leafy greens. This is due to mutations with the MTHFR allele A1298C. Folate is required for proper mitochondrial function, among other things.
17. On the cellular level, undigested proteins cause the red blood cells to become sticky and create blood structures like a roll of coins; undigested meat and gluten create plaque buildup in the artery walls.
18. Undigested proteins and plaque buildup cause significant blood sugar and blood flow issues.
19. The blood is impacted by the leaky gut as well as harmful free radicals, such as bad bacteria, Candida/fungi, parasites, and viruses, and cell debris, such as microplastics and toxic heavy metals.
20. The underlying genetic causes of all chronic illnesses are mutations or deletions within the body's lipid metabolism, bone density, insulin regulation, methylation, inflammation, detoxification, and/or oxidative stress gene groups.
21. Mutations or deletions within these key gene groups will impact the molecules and enzymes that play critical roles in various physiological processes, ensuring the proper functioning of cells and overall health.

CHAPTER 1: EXPOSURE TO TOXINS

Legal Disclaimer: This book is intended solely for informational and educational purposes. The information provided is not meant to be interpreted as medical advice or to replace the guidance of a qualified healthcare practitioner. It is imperative to consult with your provider before implementing any detoxification practices mentioned in this book. Detoxing without proper advisement from can lead to Herxing symptoms, which may include exacerbation of existing symptoms, flu-like symptoms, fatigue, headaches, muscle and joint pain, and or other adverse reactions. Herxing occurs when the body can't effectively respond to the release of toxins.

The human body is equipped with an intricate system of detoxification mechanisms designed to rid itself of harmful substances and waste products. Through key physiological processes the body continually works to eliminate toxins and maintain internal balance.

The sweat glands, kidneys, digestive system, lungs, and brain all play crucial roles in detoxification process. Understanding how these mechanisms function illustrates the body's remarkable ability to cleanse and renew itself, promoting optimal health and well-being.

Here's how the body detoxes:

- Sweat: This is a natural process by which the body releases toxins through the pores of the skin. When the body overheats or during physical activity, sweat glands are activated, allowing toxins, such as heavy metals and alcohol, to be expelled through perspiration.

- Urination: The kidneys play a crucial role in filtering waste products and excess substances from the blood to form urine. Urination is the body's way of eliminating these toxins, including urea, excess salts, and water-soluble toxins. Drinking plenty of water helps flush out toxins more effectively.

- Bowel movement: The digestive system breaks down food and absorbs nutrients while eliminating waste products through bowel movements. The colon, or large intestine, is responsible for the final stage of waste elimination. Regular bowel movements are essential for removing toxins, undigested food particles, and harmful bacteria from the body.

- Breathing: Through respiration, the lungs take in oxygen and expel carbon dioxide, along with other volatile organic compounds and toxins. Deep breathing exercises, such as meditation or yoga, can enhance lung function and aid in expelling toxins from the body.

- Sleep: During sleep, the body undergoes various physiological processes that promote detoxification and repair. The body's lymphatic system removes waste products, including toxins and metabolic byproducts, while cells repair and regenerate. Adequate sleep duration and quality are crucial for optimal detoxification and overall health.

△△△

We are exposed to am onslaught of toxins from various sources, including food, water, personal-care products, cookware, medications, medical testing, clothing, shoes, and air pollution.

While it is challenging to quantify the exact number of toxins encountered daily, it is estimated by watchdog groups, such as the Environmental Work Group, that the average person may be exposed to hundreds of different chemicals and contaminants daily.

The body's ability to detoxify and eliminate toxins varies depending on factors such as, toxin type, exposure level, individual health status, and detoxification capacity. Flushing accumulated toxins may take weeks, months, or years depending on the extent of exposure and the efficacy of detoxification efforts.

By adopting a non-toxic lifestyle, minimizing exposure to harmful substances, and supporting the body's natural detoxification pathways through diet, hydration, and lifestyle interventions, individuals can reduce their toxin burden and promote overall health and well-being.

Toxins are harmful substances that can negatively impact the human body's health and functionality. The human body can be exposed to toxins through various sources, including:

- Food: Pesticides, herbicides, fungicides, synthetic

additives, preservatives, heavy metals like mercury and lead, and contaminants like aflatoxins in food products can pose health risks. Detoxification time can vary depending on the toxin, ranging from days to weeks. To detoxify from food-related toxins, individuals can focus on consuming organic, whole foods, staying hydrated, and supporting liver function through nutrient-rich diets and herbal supplements.

- Water: Contaminants such as heavy metals (lead, arsenic), industrial chemicals (PCBs, PFAS), pesticides, pharmaceutical residues, and microbial pathogens may be present in drinking water sources. Detoxification time for waterborne toxins can range from days to months. To detoxify from water contaminants, individuals can invest in high-quality water filtration systems, consume clean and filtered water, and support kidney function through adequate hydration and herbal remedies like dandelion root tea.

- Bottled Water: Plastic bottles may leach harmful chemicals, such as bisphenol A (BPA), phthalates, and other plasticizers into the water, especially when exposed to heat or sunlight. Detoxification time for plastic-related toxins can vary, with some compounds persisting in the body for extended periods. To detoxify from plastic toxins, individuals can minimize plastic use, opt for glass or stainless-steel water bottles, and support liver health through detoxifying foods and supplements.

- Personal Care Products: Skincare products, cosmetics, shampoos, soaps, and fragrances often contain synthetic chemicals, parabens, phthalates, formaldehyde, and other potentially harmful ingredients. Detoxification time for personal care product toxins can range from days to weeks. To detoxify from these toxins, individuals can switch to natural and organic personal care products, perform regular skin brushing or dry brushing to promote lymphatic drainage, and support detoxification pathways through dietary and lifestyle interventions.

- Cookware: Non-stick cookware coated with perfluorinated compounds (PFCs), aluminum cookware, and utensils made from plastics or melamine may release toxins when heated. Detoxification time for cookware-related toxins can vary, with some compounds persisting in the body for extended periods. To detoxify from cookware toxins, individuals can switch to safer alternatives such as stainless steel, cast iron, or ceramic cookware and support liver and kidney function through detoxifying foods, herbal remedies, and hydration.

- Medications: Prescription drugs, over-the-counter medications, and supplements may contain synthetic additives, fillers, preservatives, and potential contaminants. Detoxification time for medication-related toxins can vary depending on the substance and individual factors. To detoxify from medication toxins, individuals should work closely with healthcare professionals to safely taper off medications when appropriate, support liver and kidney function through detoxifying foods and supplements, and consider natural alternatives when possible.

- Medical Testing: Exposure to radiation from

medical imaging tests (X-rays, CT scans) and contrast agents used in diagnostic procedures, such as gadolinium-based contrast agents (GBCAs) in MRI, can pose risks. Detoxification time for medical testing-related toxins can vary depending on the type and duration of exposure. To detoxify from medical testing toxins, individuals can support cellular repair and detoxification pathways through antioxidant-rich foods, herbal remedies, lifestyle interventions, and potentially utilizing zeolite as a binding agent for certain toxins, such as gadolinium.

- Clothing and Shoes: Synthetic fabrics, dyes, flame retardants, and waterproofing chemicals used in textiles and footwear may release toxins into the air and skin upon contact. Detoxification time for clothing and shoe toxins can vary, with some compounds persisting in the body for extended periods. To detoxify from clothing and shoe toxins, individuals can opt for natural fiber clothing and footwear, wash new clothing before wearing, and support detoxification pathways through dietary and lifestyle interventions.

- Air: Air pollution from vehicle emissions, industrial activities, combustion of fossil fuels, indoor air pollutants (volatile organic compounds, mold, radon), and tobacco smoke can expose individuals to toxins. Detoxification time for air pollutants can vary depending on the duration and intensity of exposure. To detoxify from air pollutants, individuals can improve indoor air quality through proper ventilation, use air purifiers with HEPA filters, and support respiratory health through herbal remedies and breathing exercises.

- Makeup: Conventional makeup often contains toxins like parabens, phthalates, formaldehyde, and heavy metals like lead and mercury, which can disrupt hormones, irritate skin, and pose long-term health risks. Detox by switching to natural and organic makeup brands, using natural makeup removers, implementing regular skincare routines, and seeking professional guidance for a smoother transition.

- Perfume/Colognes: Fragrances in perfumes and colognes often contain synthetic chemicals, such as phthalates, benzene derivatives, and synthetic musks, which can cause respiratory issues, allergic reactions, and hormonal disruption. Detox by opting for natural fragrances made with essential oils, limiting the use of conventional perfumes, ventilating indoor spaces, experimenting with DIY fragrance alternatives, and choosing fragrance-free personal care products to minimize exposure.

△△△

To transition to a non-toxic lifestyle and minimize exposure to toxins, you can take the following steps:

- Eat Organic: Choose organic fruits, vegetables, and animal products whenever possible to reduce exposure to pesticides, hormones, and antibiotics. Support liver and kidney function through detoxifying foods and herbal supplements.

- Filter Your Water: Invest in a high-quality water

filtration system to remove contaminants from tap water and avoid single-use plastic water bottles. Support kidney function through adequate hydration and herbal remedies like dandelion root tea.

- Use Natural Products: Opt for natural and organic personal care products, cosmetics, and household cleaners free from harmful chemicals. Support lymphatic drainage and detoxification pathways through regular skin brushing or dry brushing.

- Choose Safe Cookware: Use stainless steel, cast iron, glass, or ceramic cookware instead of non-stick and aluminum options. Support liver and kidney function through detoxifying foods, herbal remedies, and hydration.

- Mindful Medication Use: Take medications as prescribed by healthcare professionals and inquire about potential side effects and alternatives. Support liver and kidney function through detoxifying foods, supplements, and regular liver cleanses.

- Minimize Plastic Use: Avoid plastic food containers, water bottles, and utensils, and choose glass, stainless steel, or silicone alternatives. Support liver and kidney function through detoxifying foods, herbal remedies, and hydration.

- Ventilate Indoors: Ensure proper ventilation in indoor spaces to reduce exposure to indoor air pollutants and use air purifiers if necessary.

I want to share everything I know about detox, drawing from my personal journey and professional experience as a practitioner. When I received back-to-back HIV and cancer diagnoses, I realized the importance of having comprehensive information and support to navigate my health circumstances.

I'm committed to offering insights from as both patient and provider to give you the fighting chance I wish I had.

Detoxification isn't just about physical health — it's about addressing emotional, mental, and spiritual well-being as well. I hope to empower you to make informed decisions and find integrated approaches for your healing and support.

CHAPTER 2: THE DIAGNOSIS

As long as I can remember, there was a merry-go-round of tumultuous relationships that often resulted in tower moments in my life. It wasn't until my early 30s that I encountered one of the significant partnerships of my life with Reinaldo, a tortured soul bearing the weight of being HIV+. Our connection was shattered when, during a "med break," he transmitted the virus to me in December 2013. By January 2014, I was battling for my life.

The onset of my "conversion" event unfolded with a ferocity that mirrored the darkest depths of the human experience. It was the worst flu of my life that had taken residence within me – relentless chills, throbbing headaches, pervasive body aches, and an inability to retain food or water. I found myself confined to the cold bathroom floor, tethered to the proximity of the toilet, my sanctuary in the midst of this debilitating storm.

Beyond the physical pain, my inner conflict was causing fractures in relationships with close friends, family members, and coworkers. The gravity of my situation propelled me to a fight-or-flight moment. In an effort of radical self-preservation, I chose to sever ties with my past life.

I quit my job as head of global social media for a Fortune 500 recruiting company and liquidated the symbol of my stability

– my house. With the weight of my former existence shed, I embarked on a journey of renewal, seeking solace in the sun-soaked landscape of South Florida, a sanctuary where I hoped to rebuild my shattered world.

Upon arriving in South Florida in the summer of 2014, I immersed myself in a whirlwind of unhealthy chaos and instability. I was back and forth between metro Detroit and South Florida while my house was on the market to be sold. This marked my second stint in the region, having also resided here previously for a college semester at a small Catholic school and even ventured into Jacksonville for a brief period from 2010-2011 for a job.

Once in SoFlo, I nosedived into bad eating habits, drinking and partying. However, as funds began to dwindle, I shifted my focus towards finding employment. I found some temporary freelance gigs, such as writing for a small, now-defunct Haitian news magazine. They even sent me to Mexico City and Morelia to cover an Audi car launch event in 2015.

∆∆∆

In 2016, I secured an onsite marketing and sales consultant position for a small noninvasive cosmetic surgery and vein practice. Amid this new venture, I discovered that mold infested the office where I was required to be on-site most days. Fresh from recovering from my conversion event, I found myself grappling with the aftermath, yet reluctant to seek medical guidance out of fear of the revelations it might bring.

A worsening mold infection compounded my forthcoming

HIV infection. My body was thrust into a state of even greater distress. Inflammation engulfed my entire body. My top and bottom eyelids were swollen. Intense, pounding sinus headaches occurred daily. My stomach was bloated, and there was blood in my stools. Every night, I sweated my bed out. It was a machine-gun assault on my health that I had never experienced.

As my health deteriorated, my ability to go into the office diminished. I felt like I was full of toxins. Getting out of bed became increasingly challenging. The urgency to undergo HIV testing loomed, yet I hesitated until a former sexual partner disclosed a positive STI test to me in a text message. I subsequently tested negative for this STI.

Faced with the realization that my compromised immune system teetered on the edge, I grappled with the gravity of seeking the necessary testing, knowing that each moment brought me closer to confronting a harsh truth. I went to the local STI clinic for testing.

The wait was short, but it felt like hours upon hours. I had a pit in my stomach, my mind was moving a million miles a minute, and my thoughts were scattered.

"Anthony?"

I nodded at the woman holding my chart.

"Come on back."

I went back into the office.

"What's going on today?"

I explained my situation.

"OK, we are going to start with an HIV rapid test. We will know your results within 20-30 minutes."

It was another wait that seemed like days but was only 15 minutes. The nurse pricked my finger, and quickly completed the test. The nurse left, and when she returned soon after, she had my results. I knew what they would be, but I hoped I had more time before I had to face reality.

"You have tested positive for HIV."

The pit in my stomach dropped even lower, and I felt like I needed to either shit or vomit. I was struck with temporary paralysis.

"Are you OK? This isn't 100% final, but it's rare that these tests are inaccurate. I've only had a few cases where this was the case."

Tears began to stream down my face. She placed her hand on my hand.

"We will draw some blood for vials to be sent to the lab to confirm this test. It's OK. This is a manageable, livable disease with the right drugs. And the drugs today are far more effective than they were when this HIV/AIDS epidemic began in the 80s."

ΔΔΔ

Without treatment, HIV can progress to AIDS over a period of stages across several years. If you have below 200 T-cells, you have AIDS. If you move above 200, you return to HIV status. The HIV epidemic began in the early 1980s. The first recognized cases of what later became known as AIDS were reported in the United States in 1981. However, the virus likely originated in Central Africa in the late 19th or early 20th century before spreading globally.

The epidemic sparked significant public health efforts, research, and advocacy to understand and combat the disease, leading to significant advancements in treatment and prevention over the years. A second cousin of mine succumbed to the HIV/AIDS epidemic. He was the son of my grandma's sister, Rita.

When I first came out to my grandma, Carmen, as a teenager, one of her greatest fears was that I would get HIV and die like her sister's son.

"The way he died was just so horrible. I couldn't stand that for you," she told me.

Now, I had to confirm her greatest fear that I was now HIV+. It was surreal. I knew that my sickness from just a few months ago was my conversion event, but my mind couldn't accept what I knew in my heart. I was not faced with the new reality of being an HIV+ man. Everything quickly became uncertain — my health, my relationships, my career. Every aspect of my life, my whole existence, was in upheaval.

I called my grandma first.

"Hey, Ant, what's up? How is Florida?"

The paralysis hit again. I couldn't talk.

"Ant? Anthony? Are you there? What's wrong? Are you OK?

Can you hear me?" she asked, growing increasingly more frightened.

Finally, I blurted out, "I'm positive."

She replied, "Positive for what?"

I couldn't say it.

"Ant, positive for what?"

I took a deep breath, swallowed, and said, "Gram, I just tested positive for HIV. I am HIV+."

She didn't say anything for a minute or two.

"Gram, are you there?"

She asked, "Are you sure?"

I said, "Yes. I just got the test."

She replied, "Have them test you again."

I shared what the nurse told me.

She was quiet again before saying, "I love you."

The call ended. A family member staying at my grandma's house told me she didn't sleep that night. She was pacing her bedroom.

Next, I called my mom, Mary.

"See, I told you not to be with him," she said of my ex. "Look what you've got now — HIV."

I ended the call. She tried to call back a few times, but I sent her calls straight to voicemail.

After this, I called my Aunt Teresa. We are both the black sheep of the family. She gets me. I get her.

"You have it. There's nothing you can do now. We just have to deal with it. Just calm down, relax, and try not to think about this. Don't talk to your mom, and just be by yourself. That's what you need right now: time to get your thoughts right. I love you."

I listened to her advice. I went home and took a nap. I woke up with my clothes, bed, and pillow drenched in sweat. I felt different, like a new version of myself. I had a choice to either accept this and create a new life or end my life and deal with what happens after that.

My blood draw results came in a few days later to confirm the rapid test result. The clinic set me up with another doctor at a local clinic for HIV+ men. I went in for my appointment, and the doctor was kind. She was Hispanic, like me. She went through my lab work with me.

"Your T-cells are very low. If you had waited any longer, you would have been close to a critical situation," she said.

"What are T-cells?" I asked.

△△△

CD4+ T-cells, also known as T lymphocytes, are a type of white blood cell that plays a central role in the immune system. Mine were in the 20s.

They are produced in the bone marrow and mature in the thymus gland, which is where they get their name. T-cells are crucial for orchestrating the immune response to infections, cancer, and other threats to the body.

These cells are essential for adaptive immunity, which provides long-term protection against specific pathogens by generating memory cells that recognize and respond to previously encountered threats.

Dysfunction or depletion of CD4+ T-cells can lead to impaired immune responses, leaving individuals more susceptible to infections, cancer, and autoimmune diseases. HIV, the human immunodeficiency virus, primarily targets and infects T-cells.

Once inside the body, HIV attaches to CD4 receptors on the surface of these T-cells and enters them, effectively hijacking their machinery to replicate itself. As the virus replicates, it destroys the infected CD4+ T-cells in the process.

This leads to a progressive decline in the number of CD4+ T-cells in the body, weakening the immune system's ability to mount an effective defense against infections and other pathogens.

Over time, the depletion of CD4+ T-cells results in immunodeficiency, making individuals with untreated HIV/AIDS more susceptible to opportunistic infections, certain cancers, and other complications.

Additionally, the loss of CD4+ T-cells impacts the immune system's ability to regulate other immune responses, leading to chronic inflammation.

The destruction of CD4+ T-cells by HIV is a central feature of the disease. Monitoring CD4+ T-cell counts is a crucial part of managing HIV infection and guiding treatment decisions.

△△△

Approximately 1.2 million people in the United States are living with HIV/AIDS, and most are men who have sex with men, according to the most recent data from the CDC.

This figure is not just gay men; that's any man having sex with another man. The next affected group is Black Americans, followed by Hispanic Americans, who typically receive a later diagnosis, making it more difficult to treat the disease as it progresses.

According to the most recently available data from the Joint United Nations Programme on HIV/AIDS (UNAIDS), approximately 37.7 million people worldwide were living with HIV/AIDS. In 2020, there were an estimated 1.5 million new HIV infections globally. In the same year, approximately 680,000 people died from AIDS-related illnesses worldwide.

After receiving news about my T-cell count, I sunk deeper into a depression. The combined stress of the disease, my judgmental mom, and a mold-infested work environment put my body into a downward spiral.

I developed a severe sinus infection. My head was congested. My breathing was labored, and I had a nasty cough. My top and bottom eyelids became swollen. My throat was raw and restricted. It was difficult to swallow.

I went back to my doctor, who said all this was normal.

"It's just a sinus infection. This happens often when patients are first diagnosed," she told me.

My genetic testing for what medications my body would accept was back. I was compatible with five of the approximately 30 different available drugs.

The first drug she prescribed, Genvoya, my insurance company denied. We filed an appeal. The next drug she wrote for was denied.

The third: denied.

The fourth: denied.

Finally, after calling my insurance company, crying and begging for the drug I needed to save my life, they approved Genvoya.

This whole medication process took a few months. During this time, I did not have any drugs. I asked the doctors what else we could do.

She suggested the HPV vaccine, but after researching it, the side effects of it were symptoms I was already experiencing. I wasn't willing to double my pain and inflammation with a risky vaccine with possible side effects.

"What do you want us to do then?" My doctor asked.

"I don't know. Flush my body, reset and reboot my immune system," I said.

She looked at her nurse and then looked back at me and said, "We're doctors. We don't do that. You'll have to find someone in the holistic field."

She was right. US medical doctors lack the training and education in utilizing holistic and nutritional protocols for healing.

There are also regulatory and legal constraints, insurance issues, and time constraints in implementing such methods with the number of patients they treat.

In addition, the pharmaceutical industry sits on or has strong ties to the curriculum boards of most U.S. medical schools and regulatory boards.

I was getting sicker, and I could feel my soul slipping from my body. That feeling is like a high where you are conscious and aware, but everything feels and looks like a dream.

You feel like you are floating instead of walking. You feel more connected to the earth. You are becoming part of the collective consciousness, hearing and seeing things you didn't before.

I knew I had to seek out other opinions. I found a doctor who specialized in internal medicine. I told her the symptoms I was experiencing and what my HIV doctor said.

"Well, what's going on in your gut," she asked.

"I'm bloated, and I'm crapping blood," I said.

She felt around my lower abdomen.

"I want your HIV doctor to do an anal Pap smear on you. Today, I'm also going to put a scope up your nose to see if this is actually a sinus infection," she said.

She completed the scope. I started crying and thanked her.

"Thank you for listening and helping me," I said.

She put her hand on my knee, smiled, and said, "Don't worry. We are going to figure this out."

She told me that she would call to let me know about the scope in a few days.

"If it's fresh mucus, then it's something gut-related. If it's dark mucus, then it's sinus."

△△△

"It's fresh mucus. I sent my notes to your doctor for the anal Pap smear. It's something in your gut or gut-related," the internal medicine doctor told me when she called me a few days later after reviewing the scope results.

I felt some relief, but I still had anxiety about what it could actually be. An internal medicine doctor, also known as an internist, is a physician who specializes in the prevention, diagnosis, and treatment of adult diseases. These doctors are trained to provide comprehensive care for a wide range of conditions affecting the internal organs and systems of the body.

I was grateful I found her on Google. I selected her due to her fantastic reviews. Internists undergo extensive training in general internal medicine during their residency, which includes rotations in various medical specialties such as cardiology, gastroenterology, pulmonology, nephrology, endocrinology, and infectious diseases.

I called my HIV doctor to schedule an appointment. A week or so later, I went in for an anal pap smear. Also known as anal cytology, this is a screening test used to detect abnormal cells in the anus and lower rectum.

During this procedure, a healthcare provider collects cells from the lining of the anus using a small brush or swab. These cells are then examined under a microscope to identify any abnormalities, such as precancerous or cancerous changes.

Anal pap smears are typically recommended for individuals at higher risk of anal cancer, including men who have sex with men, individuals with HIV or other immunocompromising conditions, and those with a history of anal HPV infection or anal dysplasia. The test can help detect early signs of anal cancer, allowing for prompt intervention and treatment.

A few days after my anal pap smear, my HIV doctor's office called.

"Mr. Beven, we have your results. We need you to come in," the receptionist said.

"That doesn't sound good. Can you tell me at least if it's good or bad news?"

She replied, "I'm sorry. We just need you to come in."

I felt a pit in my stomach again. They were able to get me in the next day, which was a Friday.

"We have your results. I don't want you to wait any longer," my HIV doctor said. "You have two large transformation areas. These are pre-cancerous. However, due to the nature of your situation and your T-cell count being low, I must refer you out to a colorectal cancer specialist."

The pit from my stomach dropped again, and I felt not only nauseous but light-headed.

"Are you OK?" she asked.

I nodded.

"The receptionist will get you the specialist's name."

I needed to confirm that this was as bleak as it seemed. I emailed my dad's cousin, Margaret, who is a nurse, with my results. She confirmed I needed to see the specialist.

I went home and sunk into a deep and dark hole of depression. I felt cold chills, and I was going through end-of-life scenarios in my head. This type of depression can set in with a terminal illness diagnosis and is often referred to as situational depression.

Individuals facing a terminal illness diagnosis may experience a range of emotional responses, including sadness, anxiety, grief, and despair. I was experiencing all of this already, but this felt more intense and more pronounced.

It has snowballed into what I believe was major depressive disorder. I was suicidal and contemplating the best way to kill myself. Overdose of pills. A razor blade. Run my vehicle into water. Hang myself. Everything was crossing my mind.

CHAPTER 3: THE POWER

I woke up gasping for breath and soaked in sweat. Not from a nightmare but from the reality of the situation at hand. I was ready to end it all, but something inside of me wouldn't let me let go.

I texted a friend, "I think I'm going to kill myself."

She replied back, "Don't," and sent me an audio link to the book called "The Power" by Rhonda Byrne, who also wrote "The Secret."

"The Power" is a self-help book that explores the concept of harnessing the power of the universe to achieve one's desires and improve various aspects of life, including health, relationships, wealth, and happiness.

It builds upon the principles outlined in Byrne's earlier book, "The Secret," which revolves around the law of attraction. "The Power" delves deeper into how individuals can apply this law in their daily lives through gratitude, visualization, and positive thinking to manifest their dreams and goals.

I listened to the entire audiobook, and then I fell asleep. I woke up and listened to it again and then again. I probably listened to "The Power" a several times over the next few days. After this, everything in my life started to make sense. I experienced a mental transformation by reframing challenging situations, gaining new perspectives, understanding opposing viewpoints, and realizing my role in the life challenges I was experiencing.

I had to take accountability. Although my mom was harsh in what she said, she was right. I should have stopped communicating with my ex-boyfriend. He was physically and emotionally abusive. I allowed that and invited the HIV infection into my life because I couldn't set boundaries. I didn't love myself or respect myself, so I allowed a romantic partner to do the same.

I didn't lose control. I gave it away. I was doing this in every aspect of my life. I also recognized that the resources needed to solve my problems and improve my circumstances were all within my control. I had to identify the pieces of my puzzle and put them together in a way that was going to help me re-create my life — one that I deserved to live, not one that was on life support that I was still holding onto.

If my life was going to end, why not live my last days in peace and joy? I had to live like I was dying because I was. Would I allow myself to crash and burn? Or would I rise from the ashes like the phoenix in a renewal, a rebirth? I was undergoing a cycle of death, and this was my last chance for regeneration. I could overcome adversity, emerge stronger from challenges, and experience personal transformation.

There are two chapters in Rhonda's book that were instrumental to this process. The first is the chapter on manifesting wealth for stability. Without this, you can't support the other aspects of your transformation.

This chapter delves into the concept of manifesting financial abundance through the principles of gratitude, visualization, and positive thinking. It explores techniques for shifting one's mindset around money and attracting prosperity into your life. The chapter also discusses the importance of belief and taking inspired action to achieve financial goals.

The next key chapter focuses on using the power of the mind to manifest physical well-being and vitality. It discusses practices such as affirmations, visualization, and gratitude for improving health and healing the body. It also addresses the mind-body connection and how thoughts and emotions impact overall health and wellness.

I started with a self-assessment exercise by conducting a comprehensive audit of various aspects of my life, including self-esteem, job and career, romantic relationships, finances, and, most importantly, my health. By scrutinizing these key areas, I identified my strengths and weaknesses in each area to pave the way for personal growth and positive changes in my life trajectory.

△△△

I experienced a lot of childhood trauma. This shaped my perception of relationships. The scars of my past led me down a path where I found myself gravitating toward intimate partners who mirrored the dynamics of this trauma. This pattern was not a coincidence but rather a manifestation of the psychological imprint left by the abuse.

Abuse, whether emotional, physical or psychological, can profoundly impact someone's sense of self-worth, and perception of love and intimacy. I was unconsciously seeking out similar patterns of abuse in romantic relationships, perpetuating a cycle of emotional turmoil.

Recognizing and understanding the link between childhood trauma and relationship patterns was a crucial step in my healing journey, ultimately empowering me to break free from destructive cycles and cultivate healthier, more fulfilling connections.

I was a hyper child. I couldn't sit still. I was constantly bouncing off the walls. ADHD has been linked to MTHFR genetic mutations, which affect the body's ability to process folate and regulate neurotransmitters. These mutations can contribute to imbalances in dopamine and serotonin levels, impacting attention, focus, and impulse control, commonly observed in ADHD.

I had conflicts with classmates throughout elementary, middle, and high school. I also clashed with aunts, uncles, and cousins. I had to become a fighter early on, and I stood my ground. I was disrespectful, whether I started something or someone else did. I learned over the years how to hold my temper and my tongue.

In the words of comedian and actor Monique, "I respect everyone, but I over-respect no one."

My personality formed from an intense and challenging childhood, and at the center of this was mom. This was due to the dysfunction within her family dynamic.

Trauma is generational. She said that's the environment her dad, Trinidad, raised her and her siblings in. While she witnessed abuse, my grandpa never abused her, she said. Nonetheless, she lived with the fear and anxiety of it happening.

"I didn't know how to be a parent," she said during a family therapy session when I was 17.

The cycle of abuse affected me in significant ways. I attempted to kill myself by taking an overdose of my antidepressant pills as a teenager, and that landed me for a week in the mental hospital with other troubled teens.
Once I was able to drive, I was meeting men off the Internet and having random sex with them.

I was using sex as a coping mechanism to numb my feelings of worthlessness associated with the abuse, validation, and control through sex, and a self-destructive coping mechanism to manage my emotional pain and distress.

Peppered throughout this were parties, alcohol and drug use, and a nasty smoking habit. I was damaged.

△△△

The first thing to address was, by default, the relationship with my mom and all the trauma that came with that. The dysfunctional bond between her and I parlayed into issues I experienced with my career.

Because I had an issue with her authority and control, I had an issue with any supervisor at the jobs I had. Because my mom would supplement material things for physical displays of affection, I also developed a horrible spending habit, mostly on clothes and shoes.

My mom never told me she loved me, so I never loved myself and sought out toxic romanic partners. I do believe I suffered for years with undiagnosed post-traumatic stress disorder (PTSD) from the relationship with her and my exes. My motivation for life lessened. My drinking and drug use worsened over the years, and my eating habits were horrible.

But, ultimately, I was the one manifesting my own downfall. That acknowledgment was important for me to be able to move on.

There was so much baggage to unpack with from everything I decided for my survival, I needed to block her on my phone and stop all communication with her. I knew whatever I chose to do to ensure my survival would need to be exclusive of her.

She was never emotionally supportive of my life. She made me feel less than I was, so I lived my life like that. I was like a street animal, struggling and scraping to survive. But I would always go back to her. It was instinctive. No matter what happened, I always called her.

"What were you thinking? Never mind. You weren't thinking."

That was a common response from her.

The first step in any detox program is first to acknowledge the problem — of course, it was me, but the other part of my problem was her. I love my mom, but I know my mom.

I've set my boundaries with her. We interact cordially when we see each other, and we're both fine with this. She doesn't want to rehash anything from the past, and but that's OK. I've acknowledged and released my negative feelings about that situation to receive the opportunity to move on.

△△△

Next was my career. I started as a medical and health journalist, and then I transitioned into corporate America, where I worked for 12 years.

I worked in all aspects of the corporate marketing and communications functions — from advertising, branding, content writing, digital/social media, internal/employee communications, e-commerce, and media/public relations — for small, mid-sized, and Fortune 500 companies, generating business and brand awareness from business-to-consumer and business-to-business audiences.

It was challenging, and I made my way up the ranks quickly. From the roots of my childhood abuse grew a need for perfectionism, hyper-vigilance, and fear of failure.

None of this works in a corporate environment, and I proved that over and over to myself with job after job. I would achieve excellent results, but many times, it was to my own physical detriment.

I was making a nice salary but expected to "donate" hours beyond the standard 40-hour work week. I was often identified as a high performer and would have to pick up the slack of underperforming managers and direct reports.

Your health is never their concern. Once you stop delivering results, they will find a way to terminate your employment. It was very clear to me that I had to go solo and become an entrepreneur.

Then was my financial situation. I had money. I've always had money for food, water, and other essentials like rent, payment, and insurance. But I needed money to go out on my own. I needed startup funds. What was I going to start up?

I didn't know yet, but I was going to use what I learned from "The Power" to fuel the path to my destiny, my true life purpose. In the book, Rhonda discusses asking for what you want and receiving it through the law of attraction. She emphasizes the power of intention and positive thinking in manifesting desires.

She suggests that by clearly and confidently asking the universe for what you want and believing that it is already on its way to you, you can attract your desires into your life. This principle is a central theme in her book, and she explores various techniques and practices to harness the power of the universe to manifest abundance, happiness, and fulfillment.
I decided I would just request, "Universe, find me my dream job. The job I'll have for the rest of my time here. I want to be happy, successful, and fulfilled."

I spoke this out loud in my apartment. I was expecting some instant epiphany or some sign from the sky. There was nothing. I would have to wait.

△△△

Last was manifesting my health back. In "The Power" Rhonda Byrne says that you must know what you want to heal and how what you're trying to heal works (the actual mechanics). Then, during your manifestation meditations, detail everything to the T.

I had to study and learn about the immune system, which is a complex network of organs, tissues, cells, and molecules that work together to defend the body against harmful free radicals/pathogens, such as viruses, bacteria, fungi, and parasites.

Its main parts include:

- Bone Marrow: The bone marrow produces various immune cells, including white blood cells (lymphocytes, neutrophils, and monocytes) and red blood cells.

- Thymus: The thymus is a gland located in the chest where T cells, a type of lymphocyte, mature and differentiate into functional immune cells. In some spiritual and philosophical traditions, the thymus gland is considered a center of spiritual energy and vitality, influencing one's emotional and spiritual well-being.

- Lymphatic System: The lymphatic system is a network of vessels, nodes, and organs (the spleen and lymph nodes) that help filter and transport lymph fluid, which contains immune cells and waste products, throughout the body.

- Spleen: The spleen acts as a filter for blood, removing old or damaged red blood cells and trapping pathogens. It also contains immune cells that help fight infections.

- Lymphocytes: These are a type of white blood cell that plays a central role in the adaptive immune response. There are two main types of lymphocytes: B cells, which produce antibodies to neutralize pathogens, and T cells, which help coordinate immune responses and directly attack infected or abnormal cells.

- Innate Immune System: This provides immediate,

nonspecific defense against pathogens. It includes physical barriers (the skin and mucous membranes), chemical barriers (stomach acid and antimicrobial proteins), and immune cells (macrophages, dendritic cells, and natural killer cells) that detect and eliminate pathogens.

- Adaptive Immune System: This provides a specific, targeted response to pathogens based on previous exposure. It includes specialized immune cells (B- and T-lymphocytes) that recognize and remember specific pathogens, allowing for a more rapid and effective response upon subsequent encounters.

These different parts work together to detect, neutralize, and eliminate pathogens while also maintaining tolerance to self-antigens and preventing autoimmune reactions. I also had to gain a better understanding of my body. It's a machine that either breaks down or converts what it produces internally or takes in through air, food, skin, or water.

△△△

On the cellular level, various components help to maintain the proper functioning and survival of cells, tissues, and organisms. Dysfunction in any of these processes can lead to various diseases and health issues.

Here's a summary of key cellular-level functionality:

> Amino Acids: These are the building blocks of proteins. They play vital roles in protein synthesis, which is essential for tissue growth, repair, and maintenance.

- Enzymes: These are biological catalysts that facilitate biochemical reactions within cells. They speed up chemical reactions by lowering the activation energy required for the reaction to occur. Enzymes are involved in processes such as metabolism, DNA replication, and protein synthesis.

- Hormones: These are chemical messengers produced by endocrine glands and released into the bloodstream. They regulate various physiological processes such as metabolism, growth and development, reproduction, and stress response. Hormones can have widespread effects on cells throughout the body by binding to specific receptors on target cells.

- Neurotransmitters: These are chemical messengers that transmit signals between neurons (nerve cells) and other cells, such as muscle cells or glands. They play critical roles in controlling mood, behavior, cognition, and physiological functions such as muscle contraction and glandular secretion.

- Cell Signaling: Cells communicate with each other through various signaling pathways. These pathways involve the interaction of signaling molecules, receptors, and intracellular signaling cascades, ultimately leading to cellular responses. Signaling pathways regulate cell growth, differentiation, survival, and apoptosis (cell death).

- Membrane Transport: Cell membranes control the movement of substances into and out of cells. Various transport mechanisms, such as passive diffusion, facilitated diffusion, active transport, and endocytosis/exocytosis, regulate the movement of ions, nutrients, and other molecules across the cell membrane, maintaining cellular homeostasis.

- Gene Expression: Gene expression refers to the process by which information from a gene is used to synthesize a functional product, typically a protein. This process involves transcription (the synthesis of mRNA from a DNA template) and translation (the synthesis of a protein from mRNA). Regulation of gene expression is crucial for controlling cellular functions and adapting to changing environmental conditions.

△△△

After this crash course into how to radically change my circumstances, I called the office of the colorectal cancer specialist to schedule an appointment. I met with him, and he was very cool and candid about my situation — Anal intraepithelial neoplasia (AIN). This is a premalignant condition characterized by abnormal growth of cells within the lining of the anal canal.

It is considered a precursor to anal cancer. Although AIN itself is not always cancerous, it had the potential to quickly progress to this if left untreated like in my case. He said we could do typical chemotherapy or radiation. However, with my immune system being in such a weakened state, neither of those options was advisable or necessary at this point.

"We should do an acid roller treatment. It's less intensive, less invasive, and far more effective in treating transformation areas in the anus," he said.

The treatment was scheduled for a week out. It was a simple procedure. The colorectal doctor had a device that contained an acid that would burn the transformation areas out of my anal cavity. He inserted it inside of me, rolled it around for a few minutes, and the procedure was done. He said I would experience more blood in my stool over the next few days.

CHAPTER 4: THE ART & SCIENCE OF DETOX

To manifest my body back to homeostasis, I would have to "detox." That's what I kept hearing in my mind. Now, most doctors will try to downplay or discredit detoxing, but it's been around since ancient times. The concept of detoxification, or the removal of toxins and impurities from the body, has been intertwined with human history for a millennia, blending elements of both art and science.

Ancient civilizations across the globe recognized the importance of purifying the body to maintain health and vitality. One of the earliest mentions of detoxification can be found in ancient Egyptian texts, including the Emerald Tablets, attributed to Thoth, the Egyptian god of wisdom and knowledge.

While the exact content and origin of these tablets are shrouded in mystery and legend, they are believed to contain wisdom regarding alchemy, cosmology, and spiritual transformation. Thoth's teachings emphasize the purification of the body and soul to achieve higher states of consciousness and spiritual enlightenment.

In ancient Egypt, detoxification rituals were part of religious practices and healing traditions. Egyptians used various herbs, minerals, and natural substances to detoxify. They believed in the power of cleansing baths, herbal infusions, and enemas to rid the body of impurities and restore balance.

Other ancient civilization also developed their own detoxification practices, such as:

AYURVEDA

India's traditional medicine system, emphasizes detoxification through dietary changes, herbal remedies, and purification therapies like Panchakarma.

TRADITIONAL CHINESE MEDICINE

This employs acupuncture, herbal medicine, and therapeutic exercises to support the body's detoxification pathways.

GREEK AND ROMAN MEDICINE

These physicians prescribed fasting, herbal medicines, and hydrotherapy for detoxification purposes. The Greek physician Hippocrates, often referred to as the father of medicine, famously stated, "Let food be thy medicine and medicine be thy food," highlighting the importance of diet and lifestyle in maintaining health and detoxifying the body.

∆∆∆

Throughout history, detoxification practices evolved alongside advancements in medicine and scientific understanding. In modern times, detoxification has become a prominent aspect of holistic health approaches, with methods ranging from juice cleanses and fasting to saunas and colon hydrotherapy.

Overall, the art and science of detoxification have deep roots in ancient civilizations, where people recognized the interconnectedness of physical, mental, and spiritual well-being and employed various methods to cleanse and rejuvenate the body.

The transition from natural healing methods to allopathic ("conventional") medicine occurred gradually over centuries, with significant shifts occurring during the 19th and 20th centuries.

Here's an overview of both approaches:

NATURAL HEALING METHODS

This encompasses a range of traditional and holistic practices to promote health and treat illness by supporting the body's innate healing abilities.

These methods often focus on using natural remedies, lifestyle modifications, and therapeutic interventions to address the root causes of disease and restore balance to the body.

Examples include:

- Herbal medicine: Using medicinal plants and botanical preparations to prevent and treat various ailments.

- Traditional Chinese medicine (TCM): Incorporating acupuncture, herbal remedies, dietary therapy, and mind-body practices to restore harmony and balance in the body.

- Ayurveda: A holistic healing system from India that emphasizes personalized dietary and lifestyle interventions, herbal remedies, yoga, and meditation to promote health and longevity.

- Naturopathy: A system of healthcare that emphasizes the body's ability to heal itself through natural therapies such as nutrition, hydrotherapy, physical manipulation, and detoxification.

- Homeopathy: Based on the principle of "like cures like," homeopathy uses highly diluted substances to stimulate the body's self-healing mechanisms.

ALLOPATHIC MEDICINE

This type of medicine is the dominant system of healthcare in Western societies and is based on principles of diagnosis, treatment, and prevention of disease using drugs, surgery, and other interventions that directly oppose the symptoms and mechanisms of illness.

Examples include:

- Pharmacotherapy: Using pharmaceutical drugs to treat diseases and alleviate symptoms by targeting specific biochemical pathways or physiological processes.

- Surgery: Performing invasive procedures to diagnose, treat, or cure diseases by removing, repairing, or altering anatomical structures.

- Diagnostic tests: Utilizing medical imaging, laboratory tests, and other diagnostic procedures to identify the underlying causes of illness and guide treatment decisions.

- Evidence-based practice: Emphasizing scientific research, clinical trials, and peer-reviewed literature to inform medical decision-making and improve patient outcomes.

- Specialization: Allopathic medicine is highly specialized, with healthcare professionals such as physicians, surgeons, and specialists trained in specific areas of medicine.

The shift from natural healing methods to allopathic medicine was driven by advancements in medical science and technology, the rise of academic medicine and institutionalized healthcare systems, and changes in societal attitudes toward health and illness.

△△△

While allopathic medicine has made significant strides in diagnosing and treating disease, there is growing recognition of the importance of integrating complementary and alternative therapies into mainstream healthcare to provide more holistic, patient-centered care.

The Rockefeller family, particularly John D. Rockefeller, played a significant role in the development of allopathic medicine in the United States through funding and support of medical schools and research institutions.

Allopathic medicine, the mainstream practice of using

drugs and surgery to treat symptoms, has its roots in ancient Greek and Roman medicine and has evolved over centuries. John D. Rockefeller's contributions helped shape the modern healthcare system.

Doctors will also tell you that the body doesn't need to "detox" because that's what the liver, kidneys, and lymphatic system do.

If any of the genes that code the body's detox organs and systems to do what they should be doing are mutated or deleted out of a person's genetic code, then patients get sick, and they stay sick.

I can personally attest to this, and I have hundreds of clients with the same or similar genetic dysfunctions.

∆∆∆

The genes responsible for the development and function of the lymphatic system, liver, and kidneys are numerous and complex, involving multiple pathways and regulatory mechanisms.

Here's an overview:

LYMPHATIC SYSTEM

Genes involved: VEGFR3, PROX1, FOXC2, LYVE1, FLT4

Function: The lymphatic system plays a crucial role in immune function and fluid balance. It transports lymph, a clear fluid containing white blood cells, throughout the body, helping to remove toxins, waste products, and pathogens from tissues and returning them to the bloodstream. It also absorbs and transports fats from the digestive system.

LIVER

Genes involved: HNF4A, HNF1A, CYP450 family, ALB, GSTM1

Function: The liver is a multifunctional organ responsible for various essential metabolic processes. It detoxifies harmful substances, metabolizes drugs, synthesizes proteins like albumin and clotting factors, stores glycogen, produces bile for digestion, and regulates glucose, cholesterol, and fat metabolism. Glutathione S-transferase M1 (GSTM1) is also crucial for detoxification processes in the liver.

KIDNEYS

Genes involved: ACE, AGT, APOE, HNF1B

Function: The kidneys play a vital role in maintaining homeostasis by filtering blood to remove waste products and excess substances, such as urea, creatinine, and electrolytes. They also regulate blood pressure, red blood cell production (via erythropoietin), acid-base balance, and water balance by adjusting urine concentration and volume.

Together, these organs, and the genes that program them, highlight the synergies, and true wonder, behind how the human body detoxes.

Apart from lymphatic system, the liver, and kidneys, several other organs and systems play roles in the body's detoxification processes.

These include:

- Skin: This is the body's largest organ and plays a crucial role in detoxification through sweat. Sweat glands help eliminate toxins, heavy metals, and metabolic waste products from the body. Saunas and steam baths can also promote detoxification through sweating.

- Lungs: These facilitate the removal of carbon dioxide and other volatile substances from the body through respiration. Deep breathing exercises and fresh air can support lung function and aid in detoxification.

- Gastrointestinal Tract: The digestive system, including the stomach, intestines, and colon, plays a significant role in detoxification by processing and eliminating waste products and toxins from food and beverages. Fiber-rich foods, probiotics, and adequate hydration support healthy digestion and elimination.

- Lymph Nodes: In addition to the lymphatic vessels, lymph nodes act as filters, removing toxins, pathogens, and cellular waste from the lymphatic fluid. They play a crucial role in immune function and detoxification.

- Colon: The colon, or large intestine, is responsible for the final stages of digestion and the elimination of solid waste products from the body. A healthy colon is essential for efficient detoxification and maintaining overall health.

- Endocrine System: Certain endocrine organs, such as the adrenal glands and thyroid gland, produce hormones that regulate metabolism, energy balance, and detoxification processes. Hormonal balance is essential for optimal detoxification and overall health.

- Brain: The blood-brain barrier helps protect the brain from harmful substances, while the glymphatic system facilitates the removal of metabolic waste products and toxins from the brain through cerebrospinal fluid circulation.

These organs and systems work together to support natural detoxification processes, helping the body to maintain health and well-being.

Implementing lifestyle habits that support these organs such as staying hydrated, eating a balanced diet, exercising regularly, and managing stress can optimize the body's ability to detoxify efficiently.

△△△

With this knowledge, I could effectively start detoxing my body, which would also create the path to changing the trajectory of my career and finances. I was getting a life manifesting bundle — health, career, and finances — for the price of one from the universe. Yes!

But I wanted to confirm everything I was going through with someone more in touch with the spiritual realm. I Googled for a "psychic near me." I found a gypsy psychic just north of Miami.

Her reviews were legit, and if the vibes were sketchy, I would leave. It was definitely sketchy, but something told me to stay. She was working out of an old and dingy motel.

I did end up having to leave because the psychic said the energy around me wouldn't allow for a clear reading. I had to do something unusual. She gave me a clear crystal inside of a velvet pouch to carry around at all times for one week prior to my next meeting with her.

I did what she asked, and then I returned for the reading. Before the reading, she asked for the velvet pouch and took the crystal out.

She examined it and then asked, "Did you drop the crystal?"

"No, why?"

"OK, good. This means the crystal worked."

"How do you know?"

The psychic handed me the crystal. I looked into it and then handed it back. She gazed into it for a few more minutes and then pulled some cards from a tarot deck.

"You are going to be a doctor."

"Huh?" I said confusedly. "I'm a marketing executive. I'm mid-career. I'm not going back to school. I'm not going to medical school. I don't even want to be a doctor."

"This is what crystal shows and cards confirm," she said.

She was middle-aged with dyed blonde hair and looked to be in her mid-60s. She wore bright red lipstick and had a deep and raspy voice with a Romanian accent. She sounded like a heavy smoker.

"How?"

"You cure yourself. In curing yourself, you find how to cure everyone. That's what spirit guides show."

"How do you know that's even accurate?" I asked with

skepticism.

"Accurate because the energy around you is clear to read. It's crystal in a velvet pouch. A crack in the center of the crystal means negative spirits trapped to give a clear reading."

It sounded strange, but something about her words rang true.

△△△

Numerous natural methods are available to support the body's detoxification processes, ranging from dietary changes and lifestyle modifications to alternative therapies and ancient healing practices.

By incorporating these approaches into our daily routine, you can help cleanse our bodies, boost energy levels, and promote overall vitality.

Let's go through some of the ways I detoxed my body from then until now:

- Hydration: Drinking plenty of water helps flush out toxins through urine and sweat.

- Healthy Diet: Eating a diet rich in fruits, vegetables, whole grains, and lean proteins provides essential nutrients and antioxidants that support the body's natural detoxification processes.

- Fasting: Short-term fasting or intermittent fasting can give the digestive system a break and allow the body to focus on detoxification and repair.

- Herbal Teas: Certain herbal teas, such as dandelion, green tea, and ginger tea, can support liver function and aid in detoxification.

- Exercise: Regular physical activity promotes circulation, sweating, and releasing toxins through the skin. I did fast cardio and interval cardio daily.

- Sauna or Steam Room: Heat therapy through sauna or steam room sessions can help open pores and facilitate the elimination of toxins through sweat. Infrared saunas use infrared light to penetrate the skin and heat the body from within, promoting detoxification, relaxation, pain relief, and improved circulation.

- Limiting Alcohol and Caffeine: Cutting back on alcohol and caffeine consumption reduces the burden on the liver and kidneys, allowing them to detoxify the body more effectively. Caffeine can also strip the gut lining.

- Colon Cleanses: Some people opt for colon cleansing procedures or supplements to remove built-up waste and toxins from the colon. I did both.

- Chiropractic Care: This involves manual manipulation of the spine and other joints to improve alignment, reduce pain, and enhance nervous system function. Some proponents suggest that chiropractic adjustments can facilitate detoxification by improving nerve flow and circulation.

- Reducing Stress: Chronic stress can impair the body's natural detoxification mechanisms, so practicing stress-reduction techniques like meditation, yoga, or tai chi can be beneficial.

- Grounding (earthing): This involves connecting the body to the Earth's surface by walking barefoot outdoors or using grounding mats indoors. Proponents say it can reduce inflammation, improve sleep, and promote relaxation by allowing the body to absorb negatively charged electrons from the Earth.

- Ionic Detox Foot Baths: This involves placing your feet in a basin of warm water with an electrical current running through it. It can help draw out toxins from the body through the feet, improving detoxification, energy levels, and overall well-being. I'm a huge proponent of this detox method.

- Sound Healing: Sound healing involves the therapeutic use of sound waves to promote physical, emotional, and spiritual well-being. Solfeggio frequencies, such as 174 Hz, 285 Hz, 396 Hz, 417 Hz, 528 Hz, 639 Hz, 741 Hz, and 852 Hz, are believed to have specific healing properties ranging from pain reduction to spiritual growth.

- Lymphatic Brushing (dry brushing): This involves using a dry brush to gently massage the skin in long, sweeping motions towards the heart. This technique is believed to stimulate the lymphatic system, helping to remove toxins and waste products from the body.

- Magnetic Healing: This involves using magnets or magnetic fields purportedly to improve circulation, reduce pain, and promote healing. Advocates believe that magnets can influence the body's electromagnetic field and restore balance.

- Frequency Healing (vibrational healing): This

involves using specific frequencies of sound, light, or electromagnetic waves to promote healing and well-being. This approach is based on the idea that everything in the universe has a unique frequency, and by matching the frequency of a particular organ or system, it can be restored to balance and health.

- Light Therapy (phototherapy): This involves exposure to specific wavelengths of light to treat various conditions, including seasonal affective disorder (SAD), sleep disorders, and skin conditions like psoriasis. Different wavelengths of light can have different effects on the body and mind, influencing mood, energy levels, and circadian rhythms.

- Cold therapy (cryotherapy): This involves exposing the body to cold temperatures for therapeutic purposes. Cold therapy can enhance detoxification by promoting vasoconstriction, which helps flush toxins from tissues, thereby reducing inflammation and stimulating the lymphatic system, which leads to improved circulation and toxin elimination.

- Adequate Sleep: Getting enough quality sleep is essential detoxification, as it allows cells to repair and regenerate. Aim for 7-9 hours of sleep per night.

- Mindfulness and Meditation: This practice can help reduce stress levels, promote relaxation, and support overall well-being, which in turn can aid in the body's detoxification efforts.

- Proper Breathing: Techniques, such as diaphragmatic breathing or pranayama, can enhance oxygenation of the blood, improve circulation, and support the body's natural detoxification processes.

- Lymphatic Drainage Massage: This gentle massage technique stimulates the flow of lymph fluid throughout the body. By applying light pressure and rhythmic movements, lymphatic drainage massage helps to remove toxins, excess fluid, and waste products from the tissues, supporting the body's detoxification process.

- Acupuncture: This is a traditional Chinese medicine practice that involves inserting thin needles into specific points on the body to stimulate energy flow and promote balance. Proponents believe that acupuncture can help improve circulation, reduce inflammation, and enhance the body's natural detoxification processes by targeting energy channels known as meridians.

- Reflexology: This is a complementary therapy that involves applying pressure to specific points on the feet, hands, or ears, which are believed to correspond to organs and systems in the body. By stimulating these reflex points, reflexology aims to promote relaxation, improve circulation, and support overall well-being. Proponents suggest that reflexology can help facilitate detoxification by enhancing the body's natural healing processes.

- Ear Candling: Ear candling, also known as thermal-auricular therapy, involves placing a hollow candle-shaped cone made of fabric coated in beeswax or paraffin into the ear canal. The candle is lit at the opposite end, creating a vacuum that supposedly draws out earwax and impurities from the ear canal. However, scientific evidence supporting the effectiveness of ear candling for detoxification is lacking, and the practice carries risks of injury and ear damage.

- Microcurrent Therapy: This involves the application of low-level electrical currents to specific areas of the body using electrodes. The electrical currents are thought to stimulate cellular repair and regeneration, improve circulation, and reduce inflammation. Proponents suggest that microcurrent therapy can aid in detox.

△△△

Don't fool yourself into thinking detox is something simple. It's a serious undertaking. Detoxing the body is akin to peeling back the layers of an onion, revealing hidden layers of toxicity that have accumulated over time. You will get sick as your body purges, too.

This is called "herxing." Just like an onion has multiple layers, our bodies can harbor various levels of toxins from environmental pollutants, processed foods, medications, and stress.

Each layer of detoxification requires careful attention and support as we work to remove harmful substances from our system. But detoxing doesn't stop there – it's just the beginning of a journey towards rebuilding the body on every level, starting with cellular health.

By supporting our cells with proper nutrition, hydration, and lifestyle changes, we can promote vitality from the inside out. Just as each layer of the onion brings us closer to its core, each step of detoxification brings us closer to uncovering our body's innate ability to survive and then thrive.

△△△

I detoxed my body from the time of my diagnosis in May until my check-in with my HIV doctor in August 2017. I just started taking Genvoya. It's a type of medication called a fixed-dose combination (FDC) HIV treatment.

Genvoya is taken once daily. After taking Genvoya orally, the active ingredients are absorbed into the bloodstream relatively quickly.

It's important to note that the exact time it takes for any HIV medication to reach therapeutic levels in the bloodstream. This depends on several factors, such as metabolism, gastrointestinal transit time, and individual differences in drug absorption.

Nonetheless, consistent adherence to the prescribed dosing regimen is critical for ensuring that an HIV drug like Genvoya remain effective in managing the infection. I'm currently taking Biktarvy, which is a medication used for the treatment of HIV-1 infection in adults and pediatric patients weighing at least 25 kg.

Biktarvy is taken orally once daily and works by inhibiting the replication of the HIV virus, thereby reducing viral load and slowing down the progression of the disease. Biktarvy and Genvoya belong to the same category of HIV medications.

△△△

At my check-in, my doctor had the nurse draw my blood to check my levels, even though I had only been taking Genvoya for a month. She told me typically, it can take several months of being on medication before reaching undetectable viral loads, but I told her I was feeling great already. She was happy to hear this.

A week or so later, her office called with my blood results. They asked me to come in and promised there wasn't bad news to share.

"Anthony, your T-cells are at 889. That's not possible for someone to have such a significant improvement in T-cell count being on medication for such a short time," she explained during my appointment. "Are you doing something in addition to the medication? It's important to tell me everything you are doing so I can best treat the HIV."

"Yes, I am detoxing."

"How are you doing this?"

"Exactly like I said I wanted you to do."

"Can you give me some examples of what you are doing?"

"I've done ionic detox foot baths and lymphatic drainage massages. I'm eating vegan and mostly fruits — ones that are very high in antioxidants, like Soursop and Mangosteen. I'm eating bitter almonds."

"That's impossible to achieve an increase in T-cell count doing what you mentioned, I'm afraid. It's not possible."

"Well, I did. You have the before-and-after results from the lab."

She nodded in disagreement and exited the exam room.

Here were my go-to's during my flush, reset, and reboot:

- Soursop: This is also known as Graviola or Guanabana, and it is a tropical fruit native to the Caribbean, Central America, and parts of South America. It is characterized by its spiky green skin and soft, white, fibrous flesh. Soursop has a sweet and tangy flavor, often described as a combination of pineapple and strawberry, with hints of citrus. In addition to its delicious taste, soursop is believed to have various potential health benefits. It is rich in vitamins, minerals, and antioxidants, including vitamin C, vitamin B6, folate, potassium, and fiber. Some research suggests that soursop may have anti-inflammatory, antimicrobial, and anticancer properties, although further studies are needed to confirm these effects. Soursop is commonly consumed fresh or used to make beverages, smoothies, desserts, and traditional remedies in regions where it grows.

- Mangosteen: This is another tropical fruit native to Southeast Asia, particularly Thailand, Indonesia, Malaysia, and the Philippines. It is known for its dark purple or reddish-purple rind and juicy, snow-white segments of flesh inside. Mangosteen has a sweet and tangy flavor, often likened to a combination of peach, strawberry, and citrus fruits. Mangosteen is prized not only for its delicious taste but also for its potential health benefits. It is rich in vitamins, minerals, and antioxidants, including vitamin C, vitamin B6, folate, potassium, and xanthones, which are plant compounds with antioxidant properties. Some research suggests that mangosteen may have anti-inflammatory, antimicrobial, and anticancer effects, although more studies are needed to understand its health-promoting properties fully. Mangosteen is typically consumed fresh or used to make juices, jams, sauces, and herbal supplements.

- Bitter Almonds: These gained attention in the realm of natural healing due to their purported anticancer properties. Amygdalin, also known as laetrile or Vitamin B17, found in bitter almonds, was promoted as a potential cancer treatment in alternative medicine circles. It was believed that amygdalin could selectively target and kill cancer cells while leaving healthy cells unharmed. However, scientific evidence supporting the efficacy of amygdalin as a cancer treatment is limited and inconclusive. Furthermore, amygdalin poses significant health risks due to its cyanide content, and its use as a cancer treatment is not supported by mainstream medical organizations. I was only eating three once a day.

CHAPTER 5: YOUR BODY, YOUR MACHINE

Understanding human anatomy and physiology is an important step in the healing journey.

Anatomy provides knowledge about the structure and organization of the body's various parts, including bones, muscles, organs, and tissues, enabling us to comprehend the physical framework upon which physiological processes occur.

Physiology, on the other hand, explores how these structures work together to carry out vital functions, such as circulation, respiration, digestion, and nervous system communication.

By studying anatomy and physiology, we can better recognize the connections between structure and function and appreciate the complexity of biological systems.

This knowledge should serve as a foundation for healthcare professionals, researchers, and individuals alike, empowering them to diagnose and treat medical conditions, optimize health and wellness, and advance scientific understanding of the human body.

Ultimately, understanding human anatomy and physiology facilitates better health outcomes, enhances medical interventions, and fosters a deeper appreciation for the marvels of the human body.

The body functions much like a finely tuned machine, constantly converting energy and matter to sustain life or breaking down substances to eliminate waste. This process is governed by the body's genetic code, encoded within its DNA.

Just as a machine follows a set of instructions to perform specific tasks, the body's genetic blueprint dictates the formation and function of its various systems and organs.

Through the expression of genes, the body orchestrates processes such as metabolism, growth, and repair, ensuring the seamless operation of its complex machinery.

But, like any machine, the body is susceptible to wear and tear, genetic mutations, and external factors that can disrupt its functioning.

Knowledge of bodily functions empowers individuals to recognize signs of illness or dysfunction, seek appropriate medical attention, and actively participate in their own healing. This awareness fosters a deeper appreciation for the complexity and resilience of human biology, encouraging a proactive approach to lead healthier, more fulfilling lives.

△△△

Here are the major body systems, along with information on what each system does:

- Integumentary System: This system includes the skin, hair, nails, and glands. It protects the body from external factors and helps regulate temperature.

- Skeletal System: Comprised of bones and cartilage, this system provides structural support, protects internal organs, and facilitates movement.

- Muscular System: Made up of muscles, tendons, and ligaments, this system enables movement, supports posture, and generates heat.

- Nervous System: Consisting of the brain, spinal cord, and nerves, this system coordinates and controls bodily functions, including sensation and response to stimuli.

- Endocrine System: Comprising glands such as the pituitary, thyroid, and adrenal glands, this system regulates bodily functions through the secretion of hormones.

- Cardiovascular System: This system includes the heart and blood vessels, facilitating the circulation of blood throughout the body to transport nutrients, oxygen, and waste products.

- Respiratory System: Made up of the lungs, trachea, bronchi, and diaphragm, this system facilitates gas exchange, allowing oxygen to enter the body and carbon dioxide to be expelled.

- Digestive System: Comprised of organs such as the stomach, intestines, liver, and pancreas, this system processes food, extracts nutrients, and eliminates waste.

- Urinary System: Consisting of the kidneys, ureters, bladder, and urethra, this system removes waste products from the blood and regulates fluid balance and electrolytes.

- Lymphatic System/Immune System: Including lymph nodes, spleen, thymus, and lymphatic vessels, this system defends the body against pathogens and helps maintain fluid balance.
- Reproductive System: Different in males and females, this system enables reproduction through the production of gametes (sperm and eggs) and the facilitation of fertilization and pregnancy.

Each of these systems plays a vital role in maintaining homeostasis within the body. It's easy to overlook the most intricate and sophisticated machine of all: the human body.

From the rhythmic beating of the heart to the journey of neurotransmitters in the brain, our bodies are marvels of biological engineering. It's to important to understand and respect how the body functions as a finely tuned machine.

△△△

Imagine for a moment that you're driving a high-performance sports car. Just like that car, your body is equipped with an array of systems designed to keep it running smoothly and efficiently.

At the heart of it all is your cardiovascular system, which pumps blood, oxygen, and nutrients throughout your body, fueling every cell and tissue. Meanwhile, your respiratory system ensures that your cells receive the oxygen they need to produce energy while your digestive system breaks down food and extracts essential nutrients.

But the wonders of the human body don't stop there. Your nervous system serves as the body's communication network, transmitting electrical signals between your brain and every other part of your body.

Your immune system stands guard against invading pathogens, while your endocrine system regulates everything from metabolism to mood through the release of hormones.

Together, these systems work in harmony to keep you alive and thriving. Like any machine, your body requires regular maintenance and care to function optimally. Listening to your body's signals is one of the most crucial aspects of this maintenance.

Pain, fatigue, and discomfort are not just nuisances to be ignored; they're your body's way of telling you that something isn't quite right. Paying attention to these signals and addressing them promptly can prevent minor issues from snowballing into more significant problems.

Understanding your body's unique needs and limitations is key to achieving optimal health and well-being. Just as a high-performance car requires the right fuel and maintenance schedule to operate at its best, your body performs best with a balanced diet, regular exercise, and adequate sleep.

By prioritizing self-care and making informed choices about your lifestyle, you can ensure that your body continues to function as the well-oiled machine it was designed to be.

∆∆∆

In recent years, researchers have increasingly recognized the profound connection between the body and mind. Stress, anxiety, and other mental health issues can take a toll on physical well-being, just as poor physical health can impact mental and emotional resilience. As such, it's essential to adopt a holistic approach to health that addresses the needs of both body and mind.

Practices such as mindfulness meditation, yoga, and deep breathing exercises can help promote relaxation, reduce stress, and enhance overall well-being. Additionally, prioritizing hobbies and activities that bring you joy, and fulfillment can nourish your soul and contribute to a sense of wholeness and balance.

In a world that often prioritizes productivity and achievement over self-care, it's easy to neglect our bodies. By recognizing the complexity and resilience of the human body, we can cultivate a deeper appreciation for the miraculous machine that carries us through life.

Your body, your machine, serves as a reminder to honor and respect the vessel that houses our consciousness and allows us to experience the world.

By listening to our bodies, nurturing our physical and emotional well-being, and adopting a holistic approach to health, we can unlock the full potential of this extraordinary machine and live life to the fullest.

Knowledge empowers you to patients to communicate effectively with healthcare professionals about their symptoms, concerns, and treatment options.Collaborative decision-making ensures tailored care is received.

When you understand how treatments and medications work within your body, you are more likely to adhere to prescribed plans for better health outcomes. Knowledge is empowerment.

ΔΔΔ

Manifestation, particularly concerning health, is another concept often associated with mindfulness and the mind-body connection.

It's important to acknowledge that manifesting sickness or healing solely through meditation does not replace medical treatment. However, some believe that cultivating a positive mindset and utilizing visualization techniques can complement traditional healthcare practices.

Here's a breakdown of how you might approach manifesting sickness out of the body and healing in through a meditative state:

THE 369 MANIFESTATION METHOD

This method is a popular manifestation technique that involves setting intentions and affirmations to manifest desired outcomes in one's life.

It is based on the Law of Attraction, which suggests that thoughts and beliefs can influence reality and attract corresponding experiences.

Here's how it works:

- Set Your Intention: Begin by clearly defining what you want to manifest. This could be a specific goal, desire, or outcome that you wish to achieve. It's essential to be specific and focused on what you truly desire.

- Write Affirmations: Write down your affirmations or intentions in the present tense as if they have already manifested. Keep your affirmations positive, empowering, and specific. For example, instead of saying, "I want to be wealthy," you would say, "I am abundant and prosperous in all areas of my life."

- Repeat Daily: Set aside time each day to repeat your affirmations. The 369 method involves repeating your affirmations three times in the morning, six times in the afternoon, and nine times at night. This repetition helps reinforce your intentions and aligns your subconscious mind with your desires.

- Visualize: As you repeat your affirmations, visualize yourself already experiencing your desired outcomes. Imagine how it feels, looks, and sounds to have manifested what you want. Engage your senses and immerse yourself in the experience as if it were already real.

- Stay Consistent: Consistency is key when practicing the 369 manifestation method. Make it a daily habit to repeat your affirmations and visualize your goals. Trust in the process and remain open to receiving your manifestations in divine timing.

- Release Attachment: Let go of any attachment to the outcome and trust that the universe will deliver what is in alignment with your highest good. Detach from the how and when of manifestation and instead focus on maintaining a positive mindset and vibration.

The 369 manifestation method can be a powerful tool for

manifesting your desires when practiced with intention, consistency, and belief. It helps to shift your mindset, raise your vibration, and align your energy with the reality you wish to create.

Here's how to manifest healing state-of-mind using this method:

- Awareness: Begin by becoming aware of any physical discomfort or symptoms present in your body. Acknowledge these sensations without judgment.

- Release Negative Energy: Through deep breathing and mindfulness meditation, focus on releasing any negative or stagnant energy associated with illness from your body. Visualize this energy dissipating with each exhale.

- Visualization: Envision yourself surrounded by healing light or energy. Visualize this energy penetrating your body and gently flushing out any toxins or illness, leaving you feeling cleansed and revitalized.

- Affirmations: Repeat positive affirmations or mantras that affirm your health and well-being. For example, "I am healthy and vibrant," or "My body is capable of healing itself."

- Gratitude: Express gratitude for your body's ability to heal and for the support of any healthcare professionals or resources available to you. Cultivating gratitude can help shift your focus away from illness and towards healing.

Here's how to further apply this method:

- Positive Intentions: Set positive intentions for your

healing journey. Focus on the outcome you desire, such as restored health, vitality, and well-being.

- Body Scan Meditation: Practice a body scan meditation, directing your attention to each part of your body and sending healing energy to any areas of discomfort or illness. Visualize these areas becoming stronger and healthier with each breath.

- Self-Compassion: Cultivate self-compassion and kindness towards yourself as you navigate the healing process. Treat yourself with the same care and gentleness you would offer to a loved one in need.

- Trust and Surrender: Trust in your body's innate ability to heal itself and surrender to the natural flow of the healing process. Let go of any fears or doubts and allow healing to unfold at its own pace.

It's important to approach these practices with an open mind and a willingness to explore their potential benefits, while not discounting traditional healing methods.

CHAPTER 6: DETOX DAY SPA

"Show me how to save my life, and I'll live my life for you." That's the karmic agreement — the deal — I put out into the universe. It responded with, first, knowledge about enzymes.

I immediately needed enzyme functionality back, I heard. I consumed copious amounts of fruits and other foods with high enzyme content, including pineapple, papaya, mango, avocado, kiwi, fermented foods (sauerkraut, kimchi, kefir, yogurt), sprouted grains, and seeds (pepitas, lentils, almonds).

After more research, I also took enzyme supplements and probiotics with prebiotics. I did anti-parasitics. I did ionic detox foot baths, lymphatic drainage massages, and used an infrared sauna. I was sweating, but feeling revitalized, not drained out of my life force. Infrared saunas penetrate beyond the surface layers of the skin, reaching deep into the body's cells to promote detoxification and cellular renewal.

I didn't know this at the time, but I was experiencing the phenomenon known as consciousness transfer. Some mystical traditions emphasize the interconnectedness of all beings and phenomena within a unified field of consciousness. This is a merging or expansion of individual consciousness into the greater cosmic consciousness, transcending the limitations of individual identity.

In the belief system of reincarnation, consciousness transfer may be understood as the soul transitioning from one physical body to another across different lifetimes. This process is often seen as part of a soul's evolutionary journey toward enlightenment or spiritual growth.

Both were happening to me. It was like the gypsy psycho said, "You are going to become a doctor." I had to be willing to let go of who I thought I was to become who I was meant to be — a healer. Someone who inspires and ignites healing within others.

I started my spa in August 2017 after receiving signs from the universe that the door was closed on corporate America. I had offers to step back into executive marketing roles, but none of them felt right.

I opened Detox Day Spa as a retail storefront after hearing those words repeatedly in my head while driving, showering, and having conversations with people. "Alright, you want me to open a detox spa," I said to the universe. I found a location near an outlet mall in the northern Detroit suburbs.

The first offering was a 90-min external detox protocol that included ionic detox foot baths, a hydromassage bed to open up the circulation, and then an infrared sauna sweat session to get the toxins out and leave with a 2.5 gallon of alkaline water to help flush and restore oxygen to the cells. It was based on my own experience.

The protocol was extremely successful. People would walk in from the street and say things like, "He wants you to know that you're doing his work," or "This place is going to thrive. I can feel it." Then they would walk out, never to return, only to deliver messages like that.

Part of manifesting my health was manifesting my destiny — to help others detox to become their own health experts as I became.

△△△

Between 2017 and 2021, I helped thousands of clients activate the healing codes within their bodies. My knowledge has helped thousands of adult, adolescent, and elderly clients either resolve or gain control of health issues related to "cancer" or severe oxidative stress, digestive discomfort, natural weight loss, parasitic infections, candida/fungal overgrowths, heavy metal toxicity, uric acid build-up, viral infections, adrenal gland concerns, hormonal imbalance, energy and sleep issues and more.

I expanded offerings to clients including live blood analysis, nutritional detox programs, microcurrent therapy, red light/blue light therapy, and DNA swab analysis.

Many have sought out my services and expertise from all around the U.S. — even the U.K. — for detox and healing on the cellular level. This includes mitochondrial dysfunction, enzyme and mineral deficiency, chronic inflammation, and oxidative stress.

Oxidative stress can be caused by harmful cell debris, like heavy metals and uric acid, and free radicals, such as parasites and Candida/fungal overgrowths.

My story and work has been featured on national TV, radio, podcasts, and news sites. I was helping so many people, and it became overwhelming. As a healer, you loan your energy to others to heal until they have the knowledge and physical capability to do it on their own. I was drained, and my body started to give way.

In May 2018, my grandma, Carmen Martinez, fell ill. She was 89, and having persistant lung infections. I remember the day I decided to take matters into my own hands and conduct a blood analysis on her.

As I peered through the microscope, what I saw shocked me – several large, multi-colored crystals comprised of both cell debris and free radicals, along with a significant lack of red blood cells. Instinctively, I knew something was seriously wrong. We rushed her to the hospital.

Once we arrived, I tried to convey my findings to the doctors, hoping they would listen and consider my observations. But, as expected, they dismissed my concerns and quickly disregarded my input. It's frustratingly common – doctors often operate in a dictatorial manner, forgetting that it's the patient's health and, ultimately, their life at stake. I had to advocate for my Gram's well-being.

I firmly requested that she be put on a magnesium and glutathione IV drips to help restore her mineral content and support her body's detox process. Yet, the doctors resisted, their egos taking precedence over collaborative patient care. It was a similar scenario with my Uncle Rudy, who battled and succumbed to prostate cancer in late 2023 after receiving several MRIs with gadolinium in contrast and several vaccinations.

In moments like these, it becomes abundantly clear that we must be our own advocates in the healthcare system. We cannot rely solely on medical professionals to make the best decisions for us. Educating ourselves, asking questions, and pushing for the treatments we believe are necessary for our health and healing is essential. My Gram was in and out of the hospital between May and just before her death on June 29.

My grandma had been my best friend, strongest supporter, and fiercest protector. I struggled to go into the spa, and I was barely eating. It was hard to grasp the fact that I had just battled my way back from the brink of near death, and now I was losing the most important part of my world. It was hard to let her go, but with the death of the old me would come a new cast of characters. I just needed to come to terms with a new reality without my Gram.

△△△

In the fall of 2018, I fell to my knees in my spa with the worst pain of my life. It was stabbing pain shooting from the left posterior part of my abdomen. I called my mom, who rushed me to the local ER clinic. It was a kidney stone, which is hard mineral and salt deposits that form in the kidneys or urinary tract.

They vary in size, ranging from as small as a grain of sand to as large as a golf ball. Kidney stones can be extremely painful and may cause complications if not treated promptly. There are different types of kidney stones, including calcium stones (the most common type), struvite stones, uric acid stones, and cystine stones.

The composition of the stone determines its treatment and prevention strategies. Kidney stones form when certain substances in the urine, such as calcium, oxalate, and uric acid, become concentrated and crystallize. Factors that increase the risk of kidney stone formation include dehydration, dietary factors such as high intake of oxalate-rich foods, family history, certain medical conditions (e.g., hyperparathyroidism), and certain medications.

The symptoms of kidney stones may vary depending on the size and location of the stone. Common symptoms include severe pain in the back, side, or abdomen, pain during urination, blood in the urine, nausea, vomiting, and frequent urination. Luckily, I only had stabbing back pain, and I was unable to urinate.

The doctor gave me a Nonsteroidal Anti-Inflammatory Drug (NSAID) IV of ketorolac to help relieve the pain and reduce the inflammation I was experiencing. Within a few hours and many glasses of water, I passed the kidney stone.

△△△

My personal and health obstacles didn't stop new clients from coming, many of whom were being referred by family members and friends who were doing my program and achieving amazing results.

I was fully booked with clients Tuesdays through Saturdays. Sometimes, I would even take clients on Sundays and Mondays when I was supposed to be closed for rest and relaxation, which I wasn't getting.

I felt chained to my karmic agreement, my deal, that if I didn't see and help everyone who came to heal, then my body would deteriorate again.

I was also becoming obsessed with learning everything I

could about healing the human form and helping people who doctors, and other holistic professionals had told couldn't be helped.

Everything and everyone that came my way was a challenge that I gladly accepted, even if to the detriment of my own health.

CLIENT SUCCESS STORIES:

- Coach E: Unable to regain health and manage weight post-cancer battle, he struggled with health and weight management. Through detox and coaching, I was able to help him lose 100 lbs. and improve his health markers with his primary care physician.

- Don: His wife, Deborah, brought him to me after her sister's successful body cleanse and mineral restoration after cancer treatments. He got his energy back and achieved bowel regularity with me. However, he died from cancer complications shortly after receiving the COVID-19 vaccine.

- Carl: Needed detoxification coaching after post-heart issues and wanted to shed unhealthy weight gain. He came to me after witnessing the success of my coaching with his wife and daughters for improved energy and hormonal balance. He achieved similar results.

- Megan: Sought help for detoxification from Morgellons Disease after finding one of my TikTok videos on the topic. I provided her with detox methods and nutritional support tailored to managing this energetic parasitic/arachnid infection.

- Tanja: Faced health challenges due to intentional HIV infection, experienced fatigue, bowel irregularity, and weakened immunity. In working with me, she achieved energy restoration, bowel regularity, and improved immune system function.

- Stefanie: Sought detoxification and restoration after breast implant leakage and discovery of MTHFR genetic mutations. She needed guidance on addressing genetic mutations and detox protocols. I provided personalized coaching and nutritional support tailored to her specific needs.

- Julie: Sought help after witnessing sister's successful detox from pain and inflammation post-car accident. She was diagnosed with multiple sclerosis, but we discovered severe heavy metal toxicity from working in her parent's manufacturing business for many years. She also had an untreated parasitic infection from a tick bite. It was hard for her to move her hands and even get out of bed. Today, she is functioning with much less pain and has her mobility back.

- Jez: Experienced a second battle with breast cancer after absorbing a client's cancer and sought help after seeing one of my MTHFR genetic mutation videos on TikTok. She received guidance on genetic mutations and personalized cancer coaching support that helped light the way toward her own healing.

△△△

Working with Jez inspired me to recognize the importance of supporting those who dedicate themselves to healing others. She emphasized the need for healers to prioritize their own well-being, acknowledging that only by replenishing their own energy can they effectively support others on their healing journeys.

This realization created a full-circle moment, as I understood that my role extended beyond simply helping those in need. My soul mission became clearer: empowering healers by "healing the healers."

By doing this, I could facilitate a ripple effect, allowing healers to carry forward the knowledge and insights gained from our interactions and apply them to their own healing practices, thus creating a positive impact on a broader scale.

Jez and the other client examples are among the thousands of clients I've had the privilege of helping. Each person's journey is unique, and I'm dedicated to providing personalized support and guidance to empower individuals to unlock their innate capacity for healing and regeneration.

Whether it's overcoming health challenges, addressing genetic mutations, or supporting detoxification and restoration, I'm committed to assisting clients in their quest for optimal health and well-being.

In my years as an integrated health practitioner, I've gained a plethora of knowledge:

- Everything comes down to protein, where meat or plants are inside the body, and how the body breaks down or converts it for use.
- Everyone has severe magnesium, and anxiety and heart issues are often related to this.
- Heavy metals are the cause of all pain and inflammation inside the body.

- Candida and parasites feed and breed in heavy metals, and also consume mineral content inside the body.

- Parasites are physical and energetic and can turn biological switches on and off inside the body.

- The body needs an electrical current to function properly, and that's why ionic detox foot baths are so effective in detoxing and restoration.

- Free radicals and cell debris can be passed from mother to child.

- Autism, Alzheimer's Disease, Parkinson's Disease, and Multiple Sclerosis are heavy metal toxicity, parasitic infection, Candida overgrowth, and severe magnesium deficiency from significant mutations and deletions within the afflicted individual's genetic code.

- Our skin absorbs everything, so be aware of your shower water, what you apply to your skin, and what you touch.

- It doesn't matter what you consume, only what your body can metabolize; this goes for food, water, supplements, and medications.

- For supplements to be effective, they must be whole food, cold-pressed and plant-based.

- Chronically sick people have little to no liver function.

- "Cancer" is severe oxidative stress caused by a complete systematic breakdown of the body.

- Hormonal imbalance is caused by trapped

emotions inside the body that infest the weakest organs, causing hormonal imbalance – either an overproduction or underproduction of hormones.

- The only thing the body doesn't need to convert is an enzyme.

- Despite the scientific terminology, the accessory organs are critical to the overall functionality of your body. Together, they are responsible for enzyme production, storage, functionality, and release, and you need an enzyme and a mineral cofactor for all the biochemical processes to occur inside the body.

△△△

From 2019 to 2021, I stayed extremely busy with the spa and clients. After my grandma died, I became reacquainted with someone I knew many years ago, Jose Antonio. He's not the ex who infected me with HIV, but he said his ex-partner did the same to him.

Things with him were great initially, but then they got off track. He had a lot of emotional baggage from his previous relationship and childhood. He became physically and emotionally abusive toward me.

The stress and trauma from all my personal issues were significantly impacting my health and the spa. I was losing clients because I couldn't focus. My body was giving in, and I was having night terrors and severe anxiety.

I had to seek out the help of a therapist who diagnosed me with Post-Traumatic Stress Disorder (PTSD). PTSD is a mental health condition that can develop after experiencing or witnessing a traumatic event, characterized by intrusive memories, flashbacks, avoidance behaviors, negative changes in mood and cognition, and heightened arousal and reactivity.

During this time, I also contracted COVID-19, caused by the novel coronavirus SARS-CoV-2. This is respiratory illness is characterized by a mild fever, cough, and difficulty breathing.

I also contracted shingles twice. Shingles, caused by the varicella-zoster virus (the same virus that causes chickenpox), is a painful rash that typically appears as a single stripe of blisters on one side of the body and is often accompanied by itching, burning, and tingling sensations.

△△△

By the end of 2021, my body, mind, and soul were tapped out. My lease at the spa was up, so I didn't renew it. By the beginning of 2022, I had moved to Florida again for a year to regroup and heal from everything. During this time, I rebranded my business, transitioning from Detox Day Spa to Detox Day Spa Nutritional Coaching.

This allowed me to expand my services beyond traditional spa treatments to comprehensive nutritional guidance and support. As part of this transition, I launched an online supplement store (Store.DetoxDaySpa.com) featuring a wide range of products tailored to support detoxification and overall wellness.

To enhance accessibility and convenience for clients, I developed a user-friendly platform complete with a symptom checker and categorized detoxes/cleanses alphabetically from A-Z. I also shifted my diagnostic focus from live blood analysis, previously conducted in the spa setting, to DNA testing and analysis.

Partnering with a shipping and fulfillment company, I was able to offer DNA swab kits to clients across the U.S., broadening the reach of individuals who could benefit from my services. From mid-2022 to mid-2023, I leveraged these new resources to provide virtual concierge coaching, guiding clients through personalized detoxification protocols and nutritional plans. However, despite these efforts, I faced another setback, and I fell ill once again.

I ended up getting a mold infection around May 2022 and a second more severe bout with long COVID. I lost a lot of weight, and there was a lot of blood in my stool. I moved back to Michigan just before Christmas 2023 but was very sick. I was having bloody bowel movements often with clots. I was very tired all the time.

My skin was dry, cracking and shedding. I had a bad cough. I was constantly winded, and it was hard to breathe, especially at night. I was sweating my bed out again.

"Is this it?" I asked the universe.

What worked the last time wasn't working this time. The doctors couldn't figure it out either.

"Show me again how to save my life," I said to the universe.

I heard "castor oil" in my head.

Castor oil, derived from the seeds of the castor plant (Ricinus communis), has been used for centuries for its various medicinal properties. Castor oil is known for its anti-inflammatory, antimicrobial, and healing properties, which would offer significant benefits in managing my anal bleeding.

My spiritual guides imparted a profound new revelation — they emphasized the importance of a holistic approach to healing beyond physical DNA analysis.

They introduced the concept of a DNA Trifecta comprising Physical, Spiritual, and Ancestral DNAs. This approach recognizes the interconnectedness of the body, mind, and spirit in the healing process.

Physical DNA addresses the body's needs for healing and regeneration, while spiritual DNA attends to the soul's journey toward inner harmony and fulfillment. Ancestral DNA taps into ancient wisdom and knowledge to unlock self-healing capabilities and ancestral lineage insights.

△△△

By spring 2023, my anus was healed, but I was still winded and had a lingering cough from long COVID. They stuck with me until early 2024. I was able to kick this from my body with Mullein leaf oil.

Mullein leaf oil is derived from the leaves of the mullein plant (Verbascum thapsus) maceration or extraction. This herbal oil is known for its anti-inflammatory, analgesic, and expectorant properties, making it popular in traditional medicine for treating respiratory conditions such as coughs, bronchitis, and asthma.

Mullein leaf oil is often used topically to soothe skin irritations, reduce inflammation, and promote healing. However, further research is needed to fully understand its potential benefits and mechanisms of action. My focus had been on everyone else's healing instead of my own, and I needed to know why my body was being hit with infection after infection.

I did a DNA swab analysis on myself. Five of my six MTHFR/methylation genes are mutated, and I am missing the gene that codes the liver for stage two of its detox process – blood cleansing for pre-carcinogens and environmental toxins like mold. I am of Mexican-American descent, and both of my nephews have similar mutations within their genetic codes.

My older nephew, Tristan, has cystic fibrosis, and my younger nephew, Winston, has autism. I believe my grandma passed away due to these mutations, which are passed from the maternal bloodline. While they were unable to diagnose her illness before her death, they found her lymphatic system was clogged, spots on her liver, and fluid around her heart and lungs.

Hispanics are the most impacted by the MTHFR genetic mutations, according to the CDC. This has resulted in Hispanics experiencing high rates of liver and kidney disease, coronary artery disease, and diabetes. The MTHFR gene, which has two alleles, 677CT & 1298AC, is responsible for breaking homocysteine down into another amino acid, methionine.

This amino acid is the key building block for proteins inside the body and neurotransmitters, such as serotonin, dopamine, and norepinephrine. The MTHFR gene is also responsible for converting folate to usable form inside the body, which is the key building block for new red blood cells.

CHAPTER 7: DNA & KEY GENE GROUPS

Understanding DNA and genetics is a key part of becoming your own health expert because it provides valuable insights into your unique biological makeup, health risks, and potential treatment responses.

Knowing your genetic predispositions can empower you to make informed decisions about your health, lifestyle, and medical care. It allows for personalized disease prevention, screening, and treatment approaches tailored to your individual genetic profile. It can identify genetic variants associated with an increased risk of certain diseases, allowing for proactive measures to mitigate risk factors and early detection of potential health issues.

Understanding how your genes may influence your response to medications can help healthcare providers optimize treatment plans, minimize adverse drug reactions, and improve therapeutic outcomes. Genetic information can also inform lifestyle choices such as diet, exercise, and environmental exposures, optimizing health and wellness based on individual genetic factors.

Despite the importance of genetics in health management,

many people may feel intimidated by science for several reasons:

- Genetics and genomics involve complex concepts and terminology that can be challenging to understand, especially for individuals without a background in biology or genetics.

- Genetic testing may uncover information about disease risk or susceptibility that individuals may find unsettling or anxiety-inducing, leading to avoidance or reluctance to pursue genetic testing.

- Misconceptions or misinformation about genetics, such as fears of genetic determinism or discrimination based on genetic information, can contribute to apprehension about genetic testing or exploration of genetic concepts.

- Ethical and Social Concerns: Genetic testing raises ethical and social considerations regarding privacy, consent, and the potential misuse or misinterpretation of genetic information, leading to apprehension or distrust of genetic technologies.

By increasing awareness, education, and accessing genetic testing resources, individuals can feel more empowered to engage with their genetics and take control of their health journey.

DNA, or deoxyribonucleic acid, is crucial for life as it contains the genetic instructions necessary for the development, functioning, growth, and reproduction of all known organisms. It serves as the blueprint for the body's structure and function.

DNA achieves this by encoding proteins, which are the building blocks of cells and tissues, as well as regulating gene expression, which determines when and where specific proteins are produced.

RNA, or ribonucleic acid, plays several essential roles in the process of gene expression. It serves as a messenger molecule, carrying the genetic information from DNA to the ribosomes, where proteins are synthesized in a process called translation. RNA molecules can also act as enzymes (ribozymes), or regulatory molecules involved in controlling gene expression.

The DNA codes for body systems, organs, and physiology through the expression of various genes. Key gene groups include:

- Homeobox genes: These are involved in the regulation of the body plan during development, determining the basic features of an organism's anatomy, such as the layout of body segments and the formation of organs.

- Oncogenes and tumor suppressor genes: These genes regulate cell growth and division. Mutations in these genes can lead to cancer development if the balance between cell proliferation and cell death is disrupted.

- Hox genes: Similar to homeobox genes, Hox genes play a role in the development of body structures. However, they are specifically involved in specifying the identity of body segments along the anterior-posterior axis.

- Transcription factors: These proteins regulate the transcription of DNA into RNA by binding to specific DNA sequences. They play critical roles in controlling gene expression and determining cell fate and function.

While DNA sequencing technologies have advanced significantly in recent years, the medical profession faces challenges in using DNA as a diagnostic tool due to several factors.

These include the complexity of genetic interactions, the presence of genetic variations that may not have clear clinical significance, and the need for extensive validation and interpretation of genetic findings.

△△△

Misdiagnosis in America is a significant issue, leading to a substantial number of deaths and serious harm. Exact statistics can vary, but it's estimated that tens of thousands of deaths occur annually due to misdiagnosis.

It's the third leading cause of death in America, according to a 2023 Johns Hopkins study. Misdiagnosis can lead to various types of deaths, including those resulting from delayed or incorrect treatment of serious medical conditions, such as cancer, heart disease, or infections.

Serious harm resulting from misdiagnosis can include complications from unnecessary treatments, worsening of the underlying condition due to lack of appropriate intervention, psychological distress, and financial burden on patients and their families.

Statistics associated with misdiagnosis-related harm highlight the need for improved diagnostic accuracy and patient safety measures within the healthcare system.

DNA testing can help to achieve this, and can give important insights into key gene groups. These are collections of genes that share similar functions or are involved in related biological processes.

For example, genes within the detoxification group encode enzymes involved in metabolizing and eliminating toxins from the body. Genes within the inflammation group encode proteins involved in the immune response and inflammatory processes.

Mutations are changes in the DNA sequence that can occur spontaneously or because of environmental factors such as radiation, chemicals, or errors during DNA replication. Mutations can alter the function of a gene, leading to changes in protein structure or expression.

Deletions are a type of mutation where a segment of DNA is lost or removed from a gene or chromosome. This can result in the loss of genetic information, leading to the absence or alteration of a gene's function.

Depending on the specific genes affected and the extent of the mutation or deletion, there can be significant impacts on an individual's health and development.

If you're chronically sick, you should have the following biological gene groups tested for any mutations or deletions:

METHYLATION GROUP

- Methylation refers to the addition of a methyl group (CH3) to DNA, RNA, or proteins, which can regulate gene expression and various cellular processes.

- Genes involved in methylation, such as MTHFR

(methylenetetrahydrofolate reductase) and COMT (catechol-O-methyltransferase), play a crucial role in processes like DNA repair, neurotransmitter metabolism, and detoxification.

- COMT is involved in the metabolism of catecholamine neurotransmitters, such as dopamine, epinephrine, and norepinephrine. It catalyzes the transfer of a methyl group to these neurotransmitters, regulating their levels and activity in the brain and peripheral tissues.

- COMT also plays a role in estrogen metabolism by catalyzing the methylation of catechol estrogens, which are intermediate metabolites of estrogen. This process helps to detoxify and eliminate estrogen from the body.

- Mutations or dysregulation in COMT can impact neurotransmitter balance, hormonal regulation, and detoxification processes, contributing to various health conditions.

INFLAMMATION GROUP

- Genes within the inflammation group encode proteins involved in the body's immune response and inflammatory processes.

- Examples include cytokines (e.g., TNF-alpha, IL-6), toll-like receptors (TLRs), and NF-kB (nuclear factor kappa-light-chain-enhancer of activated B cells).

- Mutations or dysregulation in inflammation-related genes can lead to excessive or prolonged inflammation, contributing to chronic inflammatory conditions such as rheumatoid arthritis, inflammatory bowel disease, and asthma.

DETOXIFICATION GROUP

- Genes in the detoxification group encode enzymes involved in the metabolism and elimination of toxins and xenobiotics from the body.

- Examples include glutathione S-transferases (GSTs) and UDP-glucuronosyltransferases (UGTs).

- GSTM1 (glutathione S-transferase mu 1) is a key enzyme involved in the conjugation of glutathione to various electrophilic compounds, facilitating their excretion from the body.

- Mutations or deletions in detoxification genes, such as GSTM1, can impair the body's ability to neutralize and eliminate harmful substances, leading to increased susceptibility to environmental toxins and chemical sensitivities.

BONE DENSITY

- Genes involved in bone density regulation influence bone formation, remodeling, and mineralization processes.

- Key genes include those encoding for collagen (e.g., COL1A1, COL1A2), vitamin D receptor (VDR), and osteocalcin (BGLAP).

- Mutations or variations in bone density-related genes can predispose individuals to osteoporosis, osteopenia, and other bone-related disorders, increasing the risk of fractures and skeletal abnormalities.

OXIDATIVE STRESS

- Genes within the oxidative stress group encode antioxidant enzymes and proteins involved in maintaining redox balance and protecting cells from oxidative damage.

- Examples include superoxide dismutase (SOD), catalase, glutathione peroxidase (GPx), and NRF2 (nuclear factor erythroid 2-related factor 2).

- Mutations or deficiencies in oxidative stress-related genes can lead to increased oxidative damage, inflammation, and cellular dysfunction, contributing to chronic conditions such as cardiovascular disease, neurodegenerative disorders, and aging-related diseases.

INSULIN SENSITIVITY

- Genes involved in insulin sensitivity influence glucose metabolism, insulin signaling pathways, and cellular response to insulin.

- Key genes include insulin receptor (INSR), insulin-like growth factor (IGF), and peroxisome proliferator-activated receptor gamma (PPARG).

- Mutations or dysregulation in insulin sensitivity-related genes can lead to insulin resistance, impaired glucose tolerance, and metabolic syndrome, increasing the risk of type 2 diabetes, cardiovascular disease, and obesity-related complications.

Mutations or deletions within any of these gene groups can disrupt normal physiological processes, leading to increased susceptibility to chronic illnesses and exacerbating existing health conditions. Understanding genetic predispositions can inform personalized healthcare strategies, including targeted interventions, lifestyle modifications, and disease management approaches tailored to an individual's genetic profile.

Most insurance companies will cover genetic testing if it's ordered by a doctor and deemed medically necessary. The test must be necessary for diagnosing, treating, or managing a specific medical condition or family history of genetic disorders.

It must also have clinical utility, meaning it provides information that will directly impact the patient's medical management, treatment decisions, or risk assessment.

Some insurance companies require preauthorization or prior approval before covering genetic testing to ensure that it meets their criteria for medical necessity.

Insurance companies may have preferred providers or laboratories they work with, and coverage may be limited to tests conducted by these providers.

Patients may still be responsible for copayments, coinsurance, or deductibles associated with genetic testing, depending on their insurance plan.

Translation: It's easier and quicker to pay out of pocket for genetic testing. As a chronic illness health coach, I can order DNA testing and work directly with clients, or consult and collaborate with primary care physicians for DNA testing and analysis.

CHAPTER 8: THE DIGESTIVE SYSTEM & ACCESSORY ORGANS

The digestive system is a complex network of organs and structures responsible for breaking down food into nutrients that the body can absorb. Here's a complete breakdown of the digestive system, including the main organs and accessory organs.

MOUTH

- The mouth is the entry point of the digestive system.
- It contains the teeth, which mechanically break down food into smaller pieces through chewing.
- Salivary glands produce saliva, which contains enzymes that begin the process of chemical digestion, breaking down carbohydrates.

PHARYNX

- The pharynx is a muscular tube that connects the mouth to the esophagus.
- It serves as a passage for food, liquids, and air.

ESOPHAGUS

- The esophagus is a muscular tube that transports food from the pharynx to the stomach through a series of rhythmic contractions known as peristalsis.
- It has a sphincter at both ends to prevent food from moving backward.

STOMACH

- The stomach is a muscular organ that stores and partially digests food.
- Gastric glands secrete gastric juice, containing hydrochloric acid and enzymes (pepsin) to break down proteins.
- The stomach's muscular contractions churn and mix food with gastric juice, forming a semi-liquid mixture called chyme.

LIVER

- The liver is the largest internal organ and has numerous vital functions.
- It produces bile, a substance that emulsifies fats, making them easier to digest and absorb.
- The liver also plays a role in detoxification, metabolism, and nutrient storage.

GALLBLADDER

- The gallbladder is a small, pear-shaped organ

located beneath the liver.
- It stores and concentrates bile produced by the liver.
- When needed, the gallbladder releases bile into the small intestine to aid in the digestion of fats.

PANCREAS

- The pancreas is a glandular organ located behind the stomach.
- It produces digestive enzymes (amylase, lipase, and proteases) that break down carbohydrates, fats, and proteins in the small intestine.
- The pancreas also produces insulin and glucagon, hormones that regulate blood sugar levels.

SMALL INTESTINE

- The small intestine is the longest part of the digestive tract and is where most digestion and nutrient absorption occur.
- It consists of three segments: the duodenum, jejunum, and ileum.
- Enzymes from the pancreas and bile from the liver and gallbladder further break down food molecules in the small intestine.
- Villi and microvilli, tiny finger-like projections lining the walls of the small intestine, increase the surface area for absorption of nutrients into the bloodstream.

LARGE INTESTINE (COLON)

- The large intestine reabsorbs water and electrolytes from undigested food material, forming feces.
- It consists of the cecum, colon, rectum, and anus.
- Bacteria in the large intestine ferment undigested carbohydrates and produce vitamins (vitamin K and some B vitamins).

RECTUM AND ANUS

- The rectum stores feces until it is eliminated from the body.
- The anus is the opening at the end of the digestive tract through which feces is expelled during defecation.

Each of these organs plays a unique and essential role in the digestive process, ensuring that nutrients are extracted from food and waste products are eliminated from the body.

However, the gut microbiome is critically important to overall health. This is a diverse community of microorganisms, including bacteria, fungi, viruses, and other microbes, which inhabit the digestive tract.

These microorganisms play crucial roles in digestion, nutrient absorption, metabolism, immune function, and overall health. Maintaining a balanced gut microbiome is essential for optimal well-being. To keep the gut microbiome balanced, you must do the following:

- Eat a diverse diet: Consuming a wide variety of fruits, vegetables, whole grains, and fermented foods promotes microbial diversity in the gut.
- Take enzyme supplements: Take digestive

enzymes before meals, proteolytic/anti-inflammatory after meals, and methyl enzymes on an empty stomach.

- Limit processed foods and sugar: High-sugar and processed foods can disrupt the balance of gut bacteria, favoring the growth of harmful microbes.

- Include probiotics and prebiotics: Probiotic foods (yogurt, kefir, and sauerkraut) and prebiotic foods (garlic, onions, and bananas) support the growth of beneficial gut bacteria. Prebiotics feed probiotics.

- Manage stress: Chronic stress can negatively impact the gut microbiome, so practicing stress-reduction techniques like meditation, exercise, and adequate sleep is important.

- Avoid unnecessary antibiotics: Antibiotics can disrupt the balance of gut bacteria, so they should only be used when necessary and as prescribed by a healthcare professional.

When the gut microbiome becomes unbalanced, a condition known as dysbiosis can occur. Dysbiosis involves an overgrowth of harmful bacteria, fungi, or other microbes, as well as a decrease in beneficial microbes. This imbalance can lead to digestive issues, inflammation, immune dysfunction, and an increased risk of various health problems.

Leaky gut syndrome, also known as increased intestinal permeability, occurs when the lining of the intestines becomes damaged or compromised, allowing harmful substances like bacteria, toxins, and undigested food particles to leak into the bloodstream. This increased permeability can trigger inflammation and immune responses throughout the body, contributing to a range of health issues, including autoimmune diseases, allergies, and chronic inflammation.

It's challenging to determine the exact number of Americans living with leaky gut, as it can be difficult to diagnose and may present with a wide range of symptoms.

This is a common condition, with many experts attributing its prevalence to factors such as poor diet, stress, medications, and environmental toxins. These same factors can significantly impact the accessory organs of the digestive system, including the liver, gallbladder, and pancreas.

Here's how each of these factors can affect these organs:

THE LIVER

- Diet: Consuming a diet high in processed foods, refined sugars, and unhealthy fats can lead to fatty liver disease, where excess fat accumulates in the liver. This condition can impair liver function over time.

- Stress: Chronic stress can increase cortisol levels, which may contribute to inflammation and oxidative stress in the liver, potentially leading to conditions such as non-alcoholic fatty liver disease (NAFLD) or liver fibrosis.

- Medications: Some medications, such as acetaminophen or certain antibiotics, can be hepatotoxic (toxic to the liver) and may cause liver damage or liver failure if taken in high doses or over prolonged periods.

- Environmental Toxins: Exposure to environmental

toxins such as pesticides, heavy metals, and industrial chemicals can burden the liver's detoxification processes, leading to liver damage and dysfunction over time.

THE GALLBLADDER

- Poor Diet: A diet high in saturated fats and cholesterol can increase the risk of gallstones, which are hardened deposits that form in the gallbladder. These gallstones can obstruct the flow of bile and lead to inflammation, infection, or even rupture of the gallbladder.

- Stress: Stress can disrupt normal digestive function and increase the risk of gallbladder attacks or exacerbate symptoms of gallbladder disease.

- Medications: Certain medications, such as hormone replacement therapy or cholesterol-lowering drugs, may increase the risk of gallstones or gallbladder dysfunction in some individuals.

- Environmental Toxins: Exposure to environmental toxins may contribute to gallbladder disease by disrupting bile production or promoting the formation of gallstones.

THE PANCREAS

- Poor Diet: A diet high in processed foods, sugars, and unhealthy fats can contribute to pancreatic inflammation and dysfunction. Chronic inflammation of the pancreas, known as pancreatitis, can lead to digestive problems, malabsorption of nutrients, and insulin resistance.

- Stress: Stress can exacerbate symptoms of pancreatitis or increase the risk of developing pancreatic disorders.

- Medications: Certain medications, such as corticosteroids or diuretics, may increase the risk of pancreatitis or worsen pancreatic function in susceptible individuals.

- Environmental Toxins: Exposure to environmental toxins, such as cigarette smoke or industrial chemicals, may increase the risk of pancreatic cancer or pancreatitis.

Poor diet, stress, medications, and environmental toxins can all impact the accessory organs of the digestive system, potentially leading to inflammation, dysfunction, and disease.

Adopting a healthy lifestyle, including a balanced diet, stress management techniques, and minimizing exposure to toxins, can help support the health and function of these organs.

The accessory organs of the digestive system, particularly the liver, gallbladder, and pancreas, play crucial roles in enzyme production, storage, functionality, and release, contributing to efficient digestion and nutrient absorption.

Enzymes are biological molecules that catalyze chemical reactions in the body, facilitating the breakdown of food molecules into smaller, absorbable components.

Here's how these organs support the production and function of three main groups of enzymes involved in digestion:

DIGESTIVE ENZYMES

- Digestive enzymes are primarily produced by the pancreas and play a key role in breaking down carbohydrates, proteins, and fats into simpler molecules that the body can absorb.

- The pancreas secretes digestive enzymes such as amylase (for carbohydrate digestion), lipase (for fat digestion), and various proteases (for protein digestion) into the small intestine.

- The liver also contributes to the production of bile, which is stored and concentrated in the gallbladder before being released into the small intestine. Bile helps emulsify fats, increasing their surface area for digestion by lipase enzymes.

PROTEOLYTIC ENZYMES

- Proteolytic enzymes, also known as proteases or proteinases, are enzymes that break down proteins into smaller peptides and amino acids.

- The pancreas produces several proteases, including trypsin, chymotrypsin, and carboxypeptidase, which are released into the small intestine to digest dietary proteins.

- These proteolytic enzymes play a crucial role in ensuring the proper digestion and absorption of dietary proteins, which are essential for building and repairing tissues in the body.

METHYL ENZYMES

- Methyl enzymes, also known as methyltransferases, are involved in various metabolic processes, including the methylation of molecules such as DNA, proteins, and neurotransmitters.

- While methyl enzymes are not directly involved in digestion like digestive and proteolytic enzymes, they play important roles in overall metabolism and cellular function.

- The liver is a major site of methyl enzyme activity, as it is responsible for numerous metabolic processes, including detoxification, hormone synthesis, and cholesterol metabolism.

The accessory organs of the digestive system work synergistically to ensure the production, storage, and release of enzymes necessary for efficient digestion and nutrient absorption.

By producing and releasing digestive enzymes into the small intestine, the pancreas facilitates the breakdown of carbohydrates, proteins, and fats.

The liver and gallbladder support fat digestion by producing and storing bile, which emulsifies fats for digestion by lipase enzymes. Additionally, while not directly involved in digestion, the liver plays a critical role in overall metabolism, including the activity of methyl enzymes involved in various metabolic processes throughout the body.

The coordinated function of these accessory organs ensures

the proper digestion and absorption of nutrients essential for maintaining health and vitality.

CHAPTER 9: CELL DEBRIS & FREE RADICALS

Cell debris refers to the remnants of dead or damaged cells that accumulate in the body. This debris can include various substances, such as proteins, lipids, nucleic acids, and cellular organelles.

Cell debris may also contain harmful compounds, such as toxic microplastics and heavy metals, which can enter the body through environmental exposure.

Toxic heavy metals, such as lead, mercury, cadmium, and arsenic, can accumulate in the body over time, often through ingestion, inhalation, or skin contact. These metals can disrupt cellular function, interfere with enzyme activity, and cause oxidative stress, leading to cellular damage and dysfunction.

Long-term exposure to toxic heavy metals has been linked to a range of health problems, including neurological disorders, cardiovascular disease, and cancer.

Microplastics are tiny particles of plastic that can enter the body through ingestion, inhalation, or skin contact. These particles can accumulate in tissues and organs, potentially causing inflammation, oxidative stress, and disruption of cellular function.

While research on the health effects of microplastics is ongoing, there is growing concern about their potential impact on human health, including their ability to act as carriers for other toxic substances and their potential to cause damage to organs and tissues.

Free radicals, such as parasites, Candida (yeast), fungi, viruses, and harmful bacteria, are microorganisms that can cause harm to the body by disrupting cellular function, triggering inflammation, and compromising the immune system.

These organisms can enter the body through various routes, including ingestion, inhalation, and skin contact, and may colonize tissues and organs, leading to infection and disease.

Parasites are organisms that live on or inside another organism (host) and obtain nutrients at the host's expense. Parasitic infections can cause a range of symptoms, including digestive disturbances, fatigue, and nutrient deficiencies, depending on the type of parasite and the affected organ systems.

Candida is a type of yeast that normally resides in the gut and other mucous membranes of the body. However, overgrowth of Candida, known as candidiasis, can occur in response to factors such as poor diet, stress, and antibiotic use. Candidiasis can lead to symptoms such as digestive issues, fatigue, skin rashes, and recurrent infections.

Fungi are microorganisms that can cause fungal infections, ranging from superficial skin infections to invasive systemic infections. Fungal infections can occur in various parts of the body, including the skin, nails, respiratory tract, and internal organs, and may cause symptoms such as itching, redness, inflammation, and fever.

Viruses are infectious agents that require a host cell to replicate and spread. Viral infections can cause a wide range of illnesses, from the common cold to more severe diseases such as influenza, HIV/AIDS, and COVID-19. Viruses can damage host cells directly or trigger an immune response that leads to tissue damage and inflammation.

Harmful bacteria, such as pathogenic strains of Escherichia coli, Salmonella species, and Staphylococcus aureus, can cause bacterial infections in various parts of the body, leading to symptoms such as fever, inflammation, pain, and tissue damage. These bacteria can produce toxins that contribute to disease development and may become resistant to antibiotics, posing challenges for treatment.

All of these pose threats to human health by disrupting cellular function, triggering inflammation, and compromising the immune system. Minimizing exposure to these harmful substances and supporting the body's natural detoxification and immune systems are essential for maintaining health and well-being.

Detoxifying the body of cell debris and free radicals can be a gradual process, often taking months or even years. This extended timeframe is because the toxicity accumulation within the body typically occurs over an extended period.

It's essential to understand that addressing this buildup may require multiple and varied types of detoxes. Expecting immediate results from a single detox regimen is not realistic. Instead, embracing a holistic approach and being patient with the process can lead to more sustainable and comprehensive detoxification outcomes.

Here's a breakdown of how each category of free radicals (pathogen) impacts the body, along with potential remedies:

PARASITES

Parasites can cause a range of symptoms depending on the type of parasite and the affected organ systems. Common symptoms include gastrointestinal disturbances (diarrhea, abdominal pain, and bloating), fatigue, weight loss, malnutrition, and fever. In severe cases, parasitic infections can lead to complications such as anemia, organ damage, and impaired immune function.

Remedies:

- Nutrition: Consuming a balanced diet of fruits, vegetables, whole grains, and lean proteins can support overall health and immune function. Some foods, such as garlic, pumpkin seeds, and papaya seeds, are believed to have anti-parasitic properties and may help reduce parasite load.

- Herbs: Certain herbs, such as wormwood, black walnut, and cloves, are commonly used in herbal medicine to combat parasitic infections. These herbs may be taken as supplements or consumed as teas.

- Supplements: Probiotics can help restore balance to the gut microbiome and support immune function. Additionally, supplements such as oregano oil and grapefruit seed extract may have anti-parasitic properties.

- Medications: Anti-parasitic medications prescribed by a healthcare professional are often necessary to treat parasitic infections effectively. These medications may include antiprotozoal drugs, such as metronidazole or tinidazole, or anthelminthic drugs, such as albendazole or praziquantel, depending on the type of parasite involved.

CANDIDA

Candida overgrowth, or candidiasis, can lead to a range of symptoms, including digestive disturbances (bloating, gas, and diarrhea), fatigue, recurrent yeast infections, brain fog, and skin rashes. In severe cases, candidiasis can contribute to systemic health issues and chronic inflammation.

Remedies:

- Nutrition: Following a low-sugar, low-carbohydrate diet can help starve Candida and reduce its growth. Focus on whole foods, lean proteins, healthy fats, and non-starchy vegetables. Probiotic-rich foods, such as yogurt, kefir, and sauerkraut, can help restore balance to the gut microbiome.

- Herbs: Certain herbs, such as oregano oil, garlic, and pau d'arco, have antifungal properties and may help combat Candida overgrowth. These herbs can be taken in supplement form or consumed as teas.

- Supplements: Probiotic supplements containing Lactobacillus and Bifidobacterium strains can help restore balance to the gut microbiome and inhibit the growth of Candida. Other supplements, such as caprylic acid and grapefruit seed extract, may also have antifungal properties.

- Medications: Antifungal medications, both topical and oral, may be prescribed by a healthcare professional to treat severe or persistent cases of Candida overgrowth. These medications may include azole drugs (fluconazole) or polyene drugs (nystatin).

FUNGI

Fungal infections can affect various parts of the body, including the skin, nails, respiratory tract, and internal organs. Depending on the type of fungus and the site of infection, symptoms may include itching, redness, inflammation, rash, difficulty breathing, and systemic illness. In severe cases, fungal infections can lead to complications such as pneumonia, meningitis, or sepsis.

Remedies:

- Nutrition: Eating a nutritious diet that supports immune function is important for preventing and managing fungal infections. Focus on foods rich in vitamins, minerals, and antioxidants, such as fruits, vegetables, whole grains, and lean proteins.

- Herbs: Certain herbs, such as garlic, oregano oil, tea tree oil, and pau d'arco, have antifungal properties and may help combat fungal infections. These herbs can be taken in supplement form or applied topically to affected areas.

- Supplements: Probiotics can help restore balance to the gut microbiome and support immune function, which may help prevent fungal infections. Other supplements, such as caprylic acid, grapefruit seed extract, and olive leaf extract, may also have antifungal properties.

- Medications: Antifungal medications, both topical and oral, may be prescribed by a healthcare professional to treat fungal infections. These medications may include azole drugs (clotrimazole or fluconazole), polyene drugs (nystatin or amphotericin B), or echinocandin drugs (caspofungin or micafungin), depending on the type and severity of the infection.

BAD BACTERIA

Bad bacteria can cause a range of health problems, including gastrointestinal infections, urinary tract infections, respiratory infections, skin infections, and systemic illness. Symptoms may vary depending on the type of bacteria and the affected organ systems but may include fever, inflammation, pain, and tissue damage.

Remedies:

- Nutrition: Eating a balanced diet that supports immune function is important for preventing and managing bacterial infections. Focus on foods rich in vitamins, minerals, and antioxidants, such as fruits, vegetables, whole grains, and lean proteins.
- Herbs: Certain herbs, such as garlic, ginger, oregano oil, and berberine-containing herbs (goldenseal or Oregon grape), have antimicrobial properties and may help combat bacterial infections. These herbs can be taken in supplement form or consumed as teas.
- Supplements: Probiotics containing beneficial strains of bacteria, such as Lactobacillus and Bifidobacterium, can help restore balance to the gut microbiome and inhibit the growth of harmful bacteria. Other supplements, such as cranberry extract, may help prevent urinary tract infections by inhibiting the adhesion of bacteria to the

urinary tract lining.

- Medications: Antibiotics are commonly used to treat bacterial infections. However, it's important to use antibiotics judiciously and only as prescribed by a healthcare professional, as overuse can contribute to antibiotic resistance and disrupt the balance of the gut microbiome.

VIRUSES

These can cause a wide range of illnesses, from the common cold to more severe diseases such as influenza, HIV/AIDS, and COVID-19. Symptoms of viral infections may include fever, cough, sore throat, runny nose, fatigue, muscle aches, and difficulty breathing. In severe cases, viral infections can lead to complications such as pneumonia, organ failure, or death.

Remedies:

- Nutrition: Eating a nutritious diet that supports immune function is important for preventing and managing viral infections. Focus on foods rich in vitamins, minerals, and antioxidants, such as fruits, vegetables, whole grains, and lean proteins.

- Herbs: Certain herbs, such as echinacea, elderberry, astragalus, and licorice root, have immune-boosting properties and may help prevent or reduce the severity of viral infections. These herbs can be taken in supplement form or consumed as teas.

- Supplements: Vitamin C, vitamin D, zinc, and selenium are important nutrients for immune function and may help reduce the risk of viral infections or shorten their duration. These nutrients can be taken in supplement form, especially during times of increased risk of exposure to viruses.

- Medications: Antiviral medications may be prescribed by a healthcare professional to treat certain viral infections, particularly those caused by influenza, herpesviruses, or HIV. These medications work by inhibiting viral replication and reducing the severity and duration of symptoms.

It's important to note that while natural remedies and supplements may help support the body's immune response and reduce the risk of infection, they should not replace medical treatment or be used as a substitute for proper medical care.

If you suspect you have a parasitic, fungal, bacterial, or viral infection, it's essential to consult with a healthcare professional for an accurate diagnosis and appropriate treatment.

Practicing good hygiene, such as handwashing and avoiding close contact with sick individuals, can help reduce the risk of infection and transmission of free radicals/pathogens.

CHAPTER 10: HEAVY METAL TOXICITY

Metals play essential roles in various physiological processes in the human body, serving as cofactors for enzymes, participating in cellular signaling, and contributing to structural components of tissues and organs.

Some metals are considered essential nutrients, meaning that they are required for proper functioning and health, while others are non-essential or toxic in excess.

Essential metals that the human body needs include iron, zinc, copper, manganese, selenium, and molybdenum. These metals play critical roles in processes such as oxygen transport (iron), immune function (zinc), antioxidant defense (copper, selenium), and enzyme catalysis (manganese, molybdenum).

Non-essential metals, such as lead, cadmium, arsenic, and mercury, are not required for physiological function and can be harmful to the body in excessive amounts. These metals can interfere with normal cellular processes, disrupt enzyme function, and induce oxidative stress and inflammation.

Heavy metal toxicity occurs when the body accumulates high levels of toxic metals, either through environmental exposure, dietary intake, or occupational exposure. Heavy metals can enter the body through ingestion, inhalation, or skin contact. Once absorbed, they can accumulate in tissues and organs, interfering with cellular function and causing damage to cells, tissues, and organs.

Heavy metals can disrupt various physiological processes, including enzyme function, DNA synthesis and repair, and cellular signaling. They can induce oxidative stress, inflammation, and cell death, contributing to the development of various health problems, including neurological disorders, cardiovascular disease, kidney damage, and cancer.

△△△

The most toxic heavy metal to the human body is gadolinium. It is a heavy metal element commonly used as a contrast agent in magnetic resonance imaging (MRI) scans to enhance the visibility of certain tissues and organs. The exact number of MRI scans conducted worldwide each year can vary, but MRI is one of the most commonly performed medical imaging procedures globally.

According to various estimates, tens of millions of MRI scans are performed annually worldwide. In the United States alone, it is estimated that over 30 million MRI scans are conducted each year.

The number of MRI scans continues to increase as technology becomes more widely available and the demand for non-invasive imaging modalities for diagnosing and monitoring medical conditions grows.

When administered intravenously, gadolinium-based contrast

agents (GBCAs) help improve the contrast between normal and abnormal tissues in MRI images, aiding in diagnosing and monitoring of various medical conditions.

Despite its usefulness in medical imaging, gadolinium can pose health risks, particularly for individuals with impaired kidney function. Gadolinium is excreted from the body primarily through the kidneys.

Still, in patients with compromised kidney function, it can accumulate in the body, leading to a rare but serious condition known as nephrogenic systemic fibrosis (NSF). NSF is characterized by the thickening and hardening of the skin and connective tissues, resulting in pain, stiffness, and mobility issues.

One of the unique properties of gadolinium is its similarity to calcium, a vital mineral that plays a key role in bone health and function. The body can mistakenly absorb gadolinium into bone tissue, where it can accumulate over time.

Gadolinium deposition in bone has been associated with various skeletal abnormalities and conditions, including gadolinium deposition disease (GDD). GDD is characterized by symptoms such as bone pain, joint stiffness, and muscle weakness, which can mimic the symptoms of bone disorders such as bone cancer. This similarity in symptoms can lead to misdiagnosis and unnecessary medical interventions.

While the exact mechanisms underlying gadolinium deposition and its effects on bone tissue are not fully understood, ongoing research aims to elucidate the long-term safety profile of GBCAs and identify strategies to minimize potential risks associated with gadolinium exposure during MRI scans.

In clinical practice, healthcare providers must carefully weigh the benefits and risks of using GBCAs in patients, particularly those with underlying health conditions, to ensure the safest and most effective imaging procedures possible.

△△△

Heavy metals are also used as binders in medications for various purposes, including improving drug stability, enhancing drug absorption, and controlling drug release.

Some of the heavy metals commonly used as binders in pharmaceuticals include:

- Iron salts, such as ferrous sulfate or ferrous fumarate, are used as binders in iron supplements and certain medications to treat iron deficiency anemia. Iron helps improve the formulation and bioavailability of the drug.

- Magnesium stearate, a magnesium salt of stearic acid, is commonly used as a lubricant and binder in pharmaceutical formulations to improve tablet cohesion and ease of manufacturing.

- Zinc stearate, a zinc salt of stearic acid, is used as a lubricant and binder in pharmaceuticals and cosmetics. It helps improve tablet disintegration and dissolution properties.

- Calcium carbonate and calcium phosphate are sometimes used as binders and fillers in pharmaceutical tablets and capsules. Calcium compounds can improve tablet hardness and stability.

- Aluminum hydroxide and aluminum phosphate

are used as binders and adjuvants in vaccines and antacids. Aluminum salts help enhance the immune response to vaccines and reduce gastric acidity in antacids.

It's important to note that while heavy metals may be used in pharmaceutical formulations, their presence is regulated by health authorities to ensure they meet health and safety standards.

Medications are derived from natural sources, including herbs, plants, and other traditional remedies that have been used for healing purposes for centuries.

Using medicinal plants and herbal preparations for health and wellness predates modern allopathic medicine and is still widely practiced in many cultures worldwide.

The active ingredients in many pharmaceutical drugs are often derived from natural sources and then modified or synthesized in laboratories to produce standardized doses and formulations. For example, aspirin, originally derived from willow bark, is now produced synthetically and widely used as a pain reliever and anti-inflammatory medication.

Herbal medicine continues to be an important component of integrative and complementary healthcare approaches, with many people incorporating herbal remedies into their wellness routines alongside conventional medical treatments. However, it's essential to use caution and consult healthcare professionals when using herbal remedies, as they can interact with medications and may not be appropriate for everyone.

Some of the other top toxic heavy metals include:

- Mercury: Found in seafood, dental amalgam fillings, and environmental pollution.
- Lead: Found in old paint, contaminated soil and

water, and certain consumer products.
- Cadmium: Found in tobacco smoke, contaminated food, and industrial emissions.
- Arsenic: Found in drinking water, rice, and seafood.

Heavy metals can enter the body through various routes, including:

- Ingestion: Consuming contaminated food, water, or beverages.
- Inhalation: Breathing in airborne pollutants or dust particles.
- Dermal Contact: Absorption through the skin from contaminated soil, water, or consumer products.

∆∆∆

Some people may have a higher susceptibility to heavy metal toxicity due to genetic factors, environmental exposure, dietary habits, and lifestyle factors. Mutations within genes involved in detoxification pathways, such as those encoding for metallothionein proteins (MTs) or glutathione-related enzymes (GSTs), may impair the body's ability to eliminate heavy metals efficiently, leading to increased susceptibility to toxicity.

Genes involved in oxidative stress response and detoxification pathways protect cells from damage and eliminate harmful substances, including heavy metals. Examples of genes involved in detoxification include:

- Glutathione S-transferase (GST) genes: GSTM1, GSTT1, GSTP1
- Metallothionein (MT) genes: MT1A, MT1E, MT2A

- NAD(P)H quinone oxidoreductase 1 (NQO1) gene

These genes encode enzymes that help neutralize reactive oxygen species (ROS) and detoxify xenobiotics, including heavy metals, by facilitating their conjugation and elimination from the body. Mutations or polymorphisms within these genes may affect individual susceptibility to heavy metal toxicity and other environmental exposures.

It's important to note that heavy metal toxicity can be passed from parent to child, particularly during pregnancy and breastfeeding. Heavy metals can cross the placenta and accumulate in fetal tissues, affecting the developing fetus. Similarly, heavy metals can be transferred to infants through breast milk, depending on the mother's exposure.

Detoxifying heavy metals from the body is a complex process that requires careful planning and implementation. While the specific duration and methods of detoxification can vary depending on individual circumstances and the level of heavy metal exposure, there are several considerations to keep in mind.

Before starting any heavy metal detoxification protocol, it's essential to consult with a qualified healthcare professional, such as a naturopathic doctor or functional medicine practitioner, who can assess your health status, recommend appropriate testing for heavy metal levels, and provide guidance on detox protocols tailored to your needs.

Identifying sources of heavy metal exposure is crucial for effective detoxification. Common sources of heavy metals include contaminated food and water, environmental pollution, dental fillings, and occupational exposures. Minimizing ongoing exposure to heavy metals is essential during the detoxification.

Chelation therapy involves administering chelating agents,

which bind to heavy metals in the body and facilitate their excretion through urine or feces.

Some commonly used chelating agents include EDTA (ethylenediaminetetraacetic acid), DMPS (2,3-dimercapto-1-propanesulfonic acid), and DMSA (dimercaptosuccinic acid). Chelation therapy should be administered under the supervision of a qualified healthcare provider.

During heavy metal detoxification, it's important to support the body with adequate nutrition to facilitate the detox process and replenish essential nutrients. This support may include consuming a nutrient-dense diet rich in antioxidants, vitamins, and minerals, as well as supplementation with specific nutrients known to support detoxification pathways, such as vitamin C, glutathione, and sulfur-containing amino acids like cysteine and methionine.

Proper hydration supports the body's natural detoxification processes, including kidney function and urine production. Drinking plenty of clean, filtered water throughout the day can help flush out toxins and promote the elimination of heavy metals from the body.

△△△

Binders are substances that attach to heavy metals in the gastrointestinal tract, preventing their reabsorption and facilitating their elimination from the body via feces. Some common binders used in heavy metal detoxification include:

- Zeolites are natural minerals with a porous structure and high surface area, which allows them to trap heavy metals and other toxins in the gastrointestinal tract.

- Pectin, a type of soluble fiber found in fruits, can bind to heavy metals and promote their elimination through the stool.
- Diatomaceous earth is a natural sedimentary rock composed of fossilized diatoms. Itsporous structure can trap heavy metals and toxins in the digestive tract.
- Activated charcoal is a form of carbon that has been treated to increase its surface area and adsorption capacity. It can bind to heavy metals and other toxins in the gastrointestinal tract and prevent their absorption into the bloodstream.
- Shilajit is a sticky substance that forms in rock layers in mountainous regions. It contains various minerals and organic compounds that may help bind to heavy metals and support detoxification.

As heavy metals are eliminated from the body during detoxification, there is a risk of depleting essential minerals. It's important to supplement with key minerals, such as magnesium, zinc, selenium, and calcium, to help maintain mineral balance and support overall health during the detox process.

Heavy metal detoxification should be approached gradually and cautiously to avoid overwhelming the body's detoxification pathways and causing adverse reactions. Depending on individual circumstances, detoxification protocols may last several weeks to several months, with periodic monitoring of heavy metal levels and overall health status.

Detoxification is a process that should be personalized

based on individual health needs and guided by a qualified healthcare professional. It's essential to listen to your body, monitor for any signs of adverse reactions, and adjust your detox protocol as needed to ensure safe and effective detoxification.

CHAPTER 11: PAIN & INFLAMMATION

Pain and inflammation are complex processes that occur in the body as part of the immune response to injury, infection, or other stimuli. At the cellular level, inflammation involves a coordinated series of events that help the body recognize and respond to potential threats, such as pathogens, damaged cells, or foreign substances.

Inflammation can be triggered by various factors, including physical injury, infection, exposure to toxins or allergens, and autoimmune reactions.

One of the most common inflammatory conditions is arthritis, which affects the joints, causing pain, stiffness, and inflammation. There are several types of arthritis, each with its own causes and treatment approaches.

Elevated uric acid levels in the blood can lead to a type of arthritis known as gout. Uric acid is a waste product that forms when the body breaks down purines, which are found in certain foods, including meat and dairy products. When uric acid levels become too high, it can crystallize and deposit in the joints, causing inflammation and intense pain, characteristic of gout attacks.

While holistic remedies focus on lifestyle modifications and natural therapies to reduce inflammation and improve joint health, allopathic treatments primarily aim to manage symptoms and slow disease progression through medications and surgical interventions. It's essential for individuals with arthritis to work closely with healthcare professionals to develop a comprehensive treatment plan that addresses their specific needs and preferences.

When tissue damage or infection occurs, immune cells such as macrophages and mast cells release signaling molecules called cytokines and chemokines. These signaling molecules recruit other immune cells to the site of injury or infection, leading to increased blood flow, swelling, and redness.

In response to cytokines and chemokines, immune cells such as neutrophils and monocytes migrate to the affected area to eliminate pathogens and remove damaged tissue. This process is known as phagocytosis. Neutrophils release enzymes and reactive oxygen species (ROS) to kill bacteria and degrade cellular debris. However, excessive production of ROS can also cause tissue damage and contribute to inflammation.

Inflammation involves the activation of various genes and signaling pathways that regulate immune responses, tissue repair, and inflammatory mediators. Specific genes and gene groups involved in inflammation include:

- Nuclear factor-kappa B (NF-κB): NF-κB is a transcription factor that regulates the expression of genes involved in inflammation, immune responses, and cell survival. Activation of NF-κB promotes the production of pro-inflammatory cytokines and chemokines.

- Interleukins (ILs) and tumor necrosis factor-alpha (TNF-α): ILs and TNF-α are cytokines that play key roles in orchestrating inflammatory responses, including the recruitment and activation of immune cells and the regulation of tissue repair processes.

- Toll-like receptors (TLRs): TLRs are cell surface receptors that recognize pathogen-associated molecular patterns (PAMPs) and activate inflammatory signaling pathways. TLR activation triggers the production of pro-inflammatory cytokines and the initiation of immune responses.

△△△

Heavy metals such as lead, mercury, cadmium, and arsenic can induce inflammation and oxidative stress in the body by disrupting cellular functions, activating immune responses, and promoting the production of pro-inflammatory mediators.

Heavy metals can activate inflammatory signaling pathways and stimulate the release of pro-inflammatory cytokines and chemokines from immune cells.

Chronic exposure to heavy metals can lead to persistent inflammation, tissue damage, and the development of chronic inflammatory conditions, such as arthritis, cardiovascular disease, and neurodegenerative disorders.

Inflammation is part of the immune response to infection, helping to eliminate pathogens and repair damaged tissue. But, chronic or excessive inflammation can contribute to tissue damage and exacerbate disease severity.

Infections that persist for long periods can induce chronic inflammation, leading to tissue damage, organ dysfunction, and an increased risk of complications.

Chronic inflammation has been implicated in the pathogenesis of various infectious diseases, autoimmune disorders, and cancers.

ΔΔΔ

Chronic inflammation is closely linked to the development and progression of cancer. Persistent inflammation can promote cancer cell proliferation, genomic instability, and tumor growth by creating a pro-tumorigenic microenvironment.

Inflammatory cytokines and chemokines produced during chronic inflammation can stimulate tumor cell proliferation, angiogenesis (formation of new blood vessels), and metastasis (spread of cancer cells to distant sites).

Infections caused by certain pathogens, such as hepatitis B virus (HBV), hepatitis C virus (HCV), Helicobacter pylori, and human papillomavirus (HPV), are known to increase the risk of developing certain types of cancer, including liver, stomach, and cervical cancer.

Pain and inflammation are complex processes that involve a cascade of cellular and molecular events orchestrated by the immune system.

Inflammation plays a crucial role in defending the body against infection and injury, but chronic or excessive inflammation can contribute to tissue damage, disease progression, and the development of chronic conditions such as cancer.

Understanding the mechanisms underlying inflammation can provide insights into potential therapeutic strategies for managing inflammatory disorders and reducing disease risk.

Both holistic and allopathic approaches offer various methods to reduce pain and inflammation, each with its own set of principles and treatments.

Holistic approaches include:

- Adopting an anti-inflammatory diet rich in fruits, vegetables, whole grains, healthy fats (omega-3 fatty acids), and lean proteins can help reduce inflammation. Avoiding processed foods, refined sugars, trans fats, and excessive consumption of red meat can also be beneficial.

- Many herbs and botanicals have anti-inflammatory properties and can be used as natural remedies to reduce pain and inflammation. Examples include turmeric, ginger, Boswellia, devil's claw, and bromelain. These herbs can be consumed as supplements or incorporated into teas, tinctures, or topical preparations.

- Certain supplements, such as omega-3 fatty acids, curcumin (the active compound in turmeric), glucosamine, chondroitin, and methylsulfonylmethane (MSM), have been shown to have anti-inflammatory effects and may help reduce pain and inflammation, particularly in conditions like osteoarthritis.

- Techniques such as yoga, tai chi, meditation, and deep breathing exercises can help reduce stress, promote relaxation, and alleviate pain and inflammation by modulating the body's stress response and promoting a sense of well-being.

- Modalities such as acupuncture, acupressure, massage therapy, chiropractic care, and hydrotherapy can help relieve muscle tension, improve circulation, and reduce pain and inflammation by targeting specific trigger points or areas of discomfort.

- Lifestyle changes such as maintaining a healthy weight, getting regular exercise, practicing good posture, getting adequate sleep, and managing stress effectively can all contribute to reducing inflammation and improving overall well-being.

Allopathic approaches include:

- Non-Steroidal Anti-Inflammatory Drugs (NSAIDs), such as ibuprofen, naproxen, and aspirin, are commonly used to reduce pain and inflammation by inhibiting the production of prostaglandins, which are mediators of inflammation. These medications are available over the counter or by prescription and can relieve conditions such as arthritis, muscle strains, and headaches.

- Corticosteroids are potent anti-inflammatory medications that are administered orally, topically, or via injection to reduce inflammation and suppress the immune response. They are often used to treat conditions such as asthma, allergic reactions, and inflammatory disorders like rheumatoid arthritis and lupus.

- Disease-Modifying Anti-Rheumatic Drugs (DMARDs) are a class of medications used to treat autoimmune diseases such as rheumatoid arthritis by suppressing the immune system and reducing inflammation. Examples include methotrexate, hydroxychloroquine, and sulfasalazine.

- Biologic drugs, also known as biologics, are a newer class of medications derived from living organisms that target specific molecules involved in the inflammatory process. Biologics are used to treat autoimmune diseases such as rheumatoid arthritis, psoriasis, and inflammatory bowel disease.

In addition to medication, allopathic approaches to pain management may include physical therapy, occupational therapy, transcutaneous electrical nerve stimulation (TENS), nerve blocks, and surgical interventions, depending on the underlying cause of pain and inflammation.

Integrating complementary therapies with conventional treatments can sometimes provide a more comprehensive and personalized approach to pain management and overall wellness.

CHAPTER 12: MOLD TOXICITY & DETOX

Experiencing mold toxicity can be incredibly daunting, and I've been down this road twice. Mold toxicity is a multifaceted infection that not only impacts the body but also takes a toll on the mind, often leaving individuals feeling overwhelmed and debilitated.

It underscores the importance of carefully assessing symptoms, seeking appropriate testing, and implementing a structured detox regimen tailored to one's physical and mental limitations to mitigate the risk of exacerbating symptoms, including Herxheimer reactions.

The journey of battling mold toxicity is often marked by a myriad of symptoms that can range from respiratory issues and fatigue to cognitive impairments and mood disturbances.

First and foremost, it is crucial to meticulously assess symptoms and seek the guidance of healthcare professionals who are well-versed in diagnosing and treating mold-related illnesses. Comprehensive testing, including environmental mold testing and mycotoxin analysis, can provide valuable insights into the extent of mold exposure and toxicity levels, facilitating informed decision-making regarding treatment and mitigation strategies.

A structured detox regimen tailored to individual needs is paramount in managing mold toxicity effectively. However, it is essential to proceed cautiously to avoid triggering Herxheimer reactions, also known as Herx reactions or Herxing.

These reactions occur when the body undergoes rapid detoxification, leading to the release of toxins into the bloodstream faster than the body can eliminate them. As a result, individuals may experience a worsening of symptoms, including flu-like symptoms, fatigue, headaches, muscle and joint pain, and cognitive impairments.

To mitigate the risk of this, a gradual and gentle detoxification approach that considers one's physical and mental limitations is imperative. This detoxification approach may involve implementing dietary changes, incorporating herbal supplements known for their detoxifying properties, and utilizing natural detox agents such as activated charcoal or bentonite clay.

Additionally, supporting immune function and enhancing detoxification pathways through lifestyle modifications, stress management techniques, and adequate hydration can help minimize the intensity of detox reactions.

Individuals must prioritize self-care and listen to their bodies throughout the detoxification process. Healing is a gradual and nonlinear journey. Seeking support from healthcare professionals, holistic practitioners, and support networks can provide invaluable guidance, encouragement, and reassurance.

△△△

Mold toxicity, a silent menace lurking in our homes and environments, poses significant health risks to millions worldwide. Mold thrives in damp and humid environments, proliferating in homes, workplaces, schools, and other indoor spaces. Inhalation, ingestion, or skin contact with mold spores and mycotoxins can trigger a range of health issues, particularly in susceptible individuals.

Estimating the exact prevalence of mold toxicity is challenging due to varying degrees of sensitivity among individuals and the nature of mold growth. Research suggests that millions of people worldwide are affected by mold-related illnesses, with symptoms ranging from mild to severe.

Mold toxicity commonly occurs in areas with high humidity levels and frequent moisture. It can manifest in diverse ways, affecting multiple bodily systems and cognitive functions. Common symptoms include respiratory issues, such as coughing, wheezing, sinus congestion, and neurological symptoms like brain fog, memory impairment, and mood disturbances. Prolonged exposure can exacerbate pre-existing conditions and contribute to chronic health problems.

Holistic approaches to managing mold toxicity focus on detoxification and immune support. This may involve dietary changes, herbal supplements, and natural detox agents like activated charcoal or bentonite clay to eliminate toxins from the body. Nutrient-rich foods, supplements, and lifestyle modifications also enhance the body's ability to combat mold-related inflammation and infections.

Allopathic remedies for mold toxicity primarily address

symptoms and underlying health issues. These may include prescription antifungal medications to treat fungal infections caused by mold exposure, as well as medications for respiratory symptoms, allergy management, and neurological issues to provide symptomatic relief while addressing mold-related health concerns.

Several types of mold commonly found indoors pose health risks to humans. Some of the most prevalent molds include:

- Stachybotrys chartarum (black mold): Known for its dark green or black appearance, black mold produces mycotoxins that can cause severe health problems, including respiratory and neurological symptoms.

- Aspergillus: This genus encompasses various species of mold, some of which produce mycotoxins harmful to humans. Aspergillus can trigger allergic reactions and respiratory infections.

- Penicillium: Often found in water-damaged buildings, Penicillium molds can produce allergens and mycotoxins, contributing to respiratory issues and allergic reactions.

Here are the holistic and allopathic remedies for each type of mold:

STACHYBOTRYS CHARTARUM (BLACK MOLD)

Holistic Remedies

- Dietary Changes: Eliminate sugar, refined carbohydrates, and processed foods from the diet to reduce inflammation. Focus on consuming organic fruits, vegetables, lean proteins, and whole grains.

- Herbal Supplements: Incorporate herbs with detoxifying properties, such as milk thistle, cilantro, and chlorella, to support liver function and toxin elimination.

Allopathic Remedies

- Antifungal Medications: Prescription antifungal drugs like fluconazole may be necessary to treat fungal infections caused by exposure to black mold.

- Symptomatic Relief: Healthcare professionals can prescribe medications for respiratory symptoms and neurological issues to provide relief while addressing underlying mold-related illnesses.

ASPERGILLUS

Holistic Remedies

- Dietary Changes: Avoid foods prone to mold contamination, such as peanuts, grains, and dried fruits. Emphasize anti-inflammatory foods like turmeric, ginger, and omega-3 fatty acids.

- Herbal Supplements: Consider natural antifungal agents such as oregano oil, garlic, and grapefruit seed extract to combat Aspergillus infections.

Allopathic Remedies

- Antifungal Medications: Depending on the severity of the infection, healthcare providers may prescribe antifungal drugs like voriconazole or itraconazole to treat Aspergillus-related conditions.

- Symptomatic Relief: Allergy medications and bronchodilators may be recommended to manage respiratory symptoms associated with Aspergillus exposure.

PENICILLIUM

Holistic Remedies

- Dietary Changes: Opt for a low-mold diet by avoiding aged cheeses, cured meats, and fermented foods. Increase consumption of fresh, organic produce, lean proteins, and gluten-free grains.

- Herbal Supplements: Support immune function and detoxification with herbs such as astragalus, echinacea, and licorice root.

Allopathic Remedies

- Antifungal Medications: Healthcare providers may prescribe antifungal medications like amphotericin B or voriconazole to treat Penicillium infections.

- Symptomatic Relief: Antihistamines, corticosteroids, and decongestants may be prescribed to alleviate allergic reactions and respiratory symptoms caused by Penicillium exposure.

△△△

Accurate diagnosis of mold toxicity involves comprehensive testing to assess environmental mold levels and evaluate individual sensitivity.

Environmental mold testing is a crucial step in identifying and assessing mold contamination in indoor spaces. It involves sampling the air, surfaces, and dust for mold spores and mycotoxins to determine the extent of mold contamination and identify potential health risks associated with exposure.

Here's more information on each aspect of environmental mold testing:

AIR SAMPLING

- Air sampling involves collecting air samples from various areas within a building using specialized equipment such as air pumps and spore traps.

- These samples are then analyzed in a laboratory to quantify the concentration of mold spores present in the indoor air.

- Air sampling can help identify the types of mold present, assess airborne mold levels, and determine if indoor mold levels exceed outdoor levels, indicating a potential mold problem.

SURFACE SAMPLING

- Surface sampling entails collecting samples from different surfaces within the building, including walls, ceilings, floors, and other visible mold growth areas.

- Depending on the surface and type of mold suspected, sampling methods may include tape lifts, swabbing, or bulk sampling.

- Surface samples are analyzed in a laboratory to identify the types of mold present and assess the extent of mold contamination on surfaces.

DUST SAMPLING

- Dust sampling involves collecting dust samples from various indoor surfaces, such as carpets, furniture, and HVAC systems.

- These samples are analyzed in a laboratory to detect the presence of mold spores and mycotoxins that may be present in settled dust.

- Dust sampling can provide valuable information about the distribution of mold spores and mycotoxins within indoor environments and help identify potential sources of mold contamination.

Mycotoxin testing helps to assess individual exposure to mold toxins and understanding the potential health risks associated with mold contamination.

Here's more information on mycotoxin testing:

METHODOLOGY

- Mycotoxin testing involves analyzing biological samples such as blood, urine, or tissue specimens collected from individuals who may have been exposed to mold.

- Various analytical techniques, including chromatography (e.g., liquid chromatography-mass spectrometry) and immunoassays (e.g., enzyme-linked immunosorbent assay or ELISA), are utilized to detect and quantify mycotoxins in biological samples.

- These methods allow for the identification and measurement of specific mycotoxins present in the body, providing insights into individual exposure levels and toxicity.

TYPES OF MYCOTOXINS

- Mycotoxins are toxic compounds produced by certain molds under favorable environmental conditions. Common mycotoxins associated with indoor mold exposure include aflatoxins, ochratoxin A, trichothecenes (e.g., deoxynivalenol, T-2 toxin), and fumonisins, among others.

- Each mycotoxin exhibits unique properties and may have varying degrees of toxicity, affecting different organ systems in the body.

It's essential to interpret mycotoxin test results in the context of comprehensive clinical evaluation and other diagnostic findings for accurate assessment and treatment.

Protecting yourself and your home against mold requires a proactive approach to moisture control and ventilation. Regular maintenance and vigilance are also key to preventing mold-related issues and promoting overall well-being.

CHAPTER 13: BLOOD CLEANSING & REBUILD

One aspect often overlooked in the quest for optimal health and vitality is the importance of blood cleansing and rebuilding. Our blood serves as the lifeline of our bodies, delivering nutrients, oxygen, and vital elements to every cell while removing waste and toxins.

The world is filled with environmental pollutants, processed foods, and stressors. Our blood can become burdened with toxins and impurities. Fortunately, through the practice of blood cleansing and rebuilding, we can rejuvenate our bodies from the inside out, unlocking newfound vitality and well-being.

In addition, gene alterations, such as those affecting detoxification genes like GSTM1, can impair the body's ability to eliminate harmful substances, increasing the risk of toxin-related health problems.

The blood plays a key role in transporting oxygen and nutrients, but it also helps regulate body temperature, maintains pH balance, and supports immune function.

Blood is produced in the bone marrow through hematopoiesis,

where stem cells differentiate into various blood cell types under the influence of growth factors and hormones.

Blood is protected by immune cells and antibodies that identify and neutralize pathogens. Blood cells relies on energy generated by mitochondria to maintain cellular integrity.

IRON

Iron plays a crucial role in the blood by serving as a key component of hemoglobin, the protein molecule in red blood cells responsible for transporting oxygen from the lungs to the body's tissues and organs. When you inhale, oxygen binds to the iron atoms in hemoglobin, forming oxyhemoglobin.

As blood circulates throughout the body, oxyhemoglobin releases oxygen to cells, allowing them to perform vital functions such as energy production. Iron is involved in synthesizing myoglobin, a protein found in muscles that stores oxygen for use during physical activity.

Thus, iron is essential for maintaining proper oxygen levels in the blood and ensuring the efficient functioning of cells and tissues throughout the body.

FOLATE

Folate, also known as vitamin B9, plays a crucial role in the blood by contributing to the production of red blood cells. It acts as fuel for the mitochondria, and is required for the synthesis of DNA, RNA, and proteins, which are essential for the growth and division of cells.

Folate deficiency can lead to impaired red blood cell production, resulting in anemia, a condition characterized by larger-than-normal red blood cells that are unable to function effectively.

Folate is also involved in the metabolism of homocysteine, an amino acid linked to cardiovascular disease, when present in high levels.

By supporting red blood cell production and regulating homocysteine levels, folate helps maintain healthy blood circulation and overall cardiovascular health.

TYPES OF BLOOD CELLS

Red Blood Cells (Erythrocytes): Transport oxygen from the lungs to the body's tissues. They contain hemoglobin, a protein that binds oxygen.

White Blood Cells (Leukocytes): Part of the body's immune system, these cells defend against infections and foreign invaders. There are several types of white blood cells:

- Neutrophils: Phagocytize bacteria and other pathogens.
- Lymphocytes: Play a key role in adaptive immunity, including B cells and T cells.
- Monocytes: Engulf and digest pathogens and cellular debris.
- Eosinophils: Involved in allergic reactions and defense against parasites.
- Basophils: Release histamine and other inflammatory mediators in response to allergens.

Top blood diseases with holistic and allopathic remedies

- Anemia: Iron-rich diet, vitamin C supplementation (holistic); Iron supplementation, blood transfusions (allopathic).

- Hemophilia: Avoidance of injury, stress management techniques (holistic); Clotting factor replacement therapy (allopathic).

- Leukemia: Nutrient-dense diet, acupuncture (holistic); Chemotherapy, bone marrow transplant (allopathic).

- Lymphoma: Immune-boosting diet, mind-body therapies (holistic); Chemotherapy, radiation therapy (allopathic).

- Thrombocytopenia: Diet rich in vitamin K, avoiding activities causing bleeding (holistic); Platelet transfusions, corticosteroids (allopathic).

- Sickle Cell Disease: Hydration, pain management techniques (holistic); Pain medications, hydroxyurea (allopathic).

- Hemochromatosis: Iron-restricted diet, regular blood donations (holistic); Therapeutic phlebotomy, iron chelation therapy (allopathic).

- Polycythemia Vera: Hydration, low-dose aspirin therapy (holistic); Phlebotomy, chemotherapy (allopathic).

- Myelodysplastic Syndromes (MDS): Nutrient-rich diet, acupuncture (holistic); Supportive care, chemotherapy (allopathic).

- Hemolytic Anemia: Diet rich in antioxidants, stress reduction techniques (holistic); Corticosteroids, immunosuppressive therapy (allopathic).

The liver metabolizes toxins and drugs, while the kidneys filter waste products and excess substances from the blood and excrete them in the urine. Burdock root can aid in blood cleansing by filtering out toxins and supporting liver function.

Blood cleansing occurs by supporting the body's natural detoxification pathways, such as the liver, kidneys, lymphatic system, and skin. Various methods can aid in blood cleansing, including dietary changes, herbal supplements, fasting, hydrotherapy, and lifestyle modifications.

Key strategies include:

- Clean Eating: Emphasize whole, nutrient-dense foods such as fruits, vegetables, whole grains, and lean proteins. Avoid processed foods, refined sugars, artificial additives, and trans fats, which can burden the liver and contribute to toxin buildup.

- Hydration: Proper hydration is essential for blood cleansing, as water helps flush toxins from the body and supports kidney function. Aim to drink at least eight glasses of water per day, and consider incorporating hydrating foods like cucumbers, watermelon, and citrus fruits into your diet.

- Herbal Support: Certain herbs possess detoxifying properties that can aid in blood cleansing. Examples include dandelion root, milk thistle, burdock root, turmeric, and ginger. These herbs can be consumed as teas, tinctures, or supplements to support liver function and enhance detoxification.

- Sweat It Out: Sweating is a natural way for the body to eliminate toxins through the skin. Engage in regular exercise, saunas, steam baths, or hot yoga to promote sweating and enhance detoxification.

- Intermittent Fasting: Periodic fasting or intermittent fasting can give the body a break from digestion, allowing it to focus on detoxification and cellular repair. Consider incorporating intermittent fasting into your routine, such as fasting for 16 hours overnight or doing a 24-hour fast once or twice weekly.

In addition to cleansing, rebuilding the blood is crucial for restoring vitality and promoting overall health. Blood rebuilding involves replenishing essential nutrients, supporting red blood cell production, and improving circulation.

Folate and resveratrol support red blood cell production and promote cardiovascular health. Colloidal copper supplements may support healthy blood flow by aiding in oxygen transport and circulation. Nitric oxide helps dilate blood vessels, improving blood flow and reducing the risk of arterial plaque buildup.

Other rebuild options include:

- Nutrient-Dense Foods: Focus on foods rich in iron, vitamin B12, folate, vitamin C, and copper, which are essential for red blood cell production and blood health. Incorporate foods such as leafy greens, lean meats, legumes, nuts, seeds, and citrus fruits.

- Iron-Rich Foods: Iron is critical to produce

hemoglobin, the protein in red blood cells that carries oxygen throughout the body. Include iron-rich foods such as spinach, lentils, quinoa, tofu, lean beef, and fortified cereals.

- Vitamin C: Vitamin C enhances iron absorption and promotes the formation of healthy red blood cells. Include vitamin C-rich foods such as citrus fruits, bell peppers, strawberries, kiwi, and broccoli.

- Herbal Tonics: Certain herbs, such as nettle, alfalfa, yellow dock, and red clover, are traditionally used to support blood health and promote circulation. Consider incorporating herbal tonics or teas into your daily routine to nourish and strengthen the blood.

- Lifestyle Factors: Prioritize adequate sleep, stress management, regular exercise, and healthy lifestyle habits to support overall blood health and vitality.

Incorporating blood cleansing and rebuilding practices into your lifestyle can profoundly affect your health and well-being. By supporting the body's natural detoxification processes, and nourishing the blood with essential nutrients, you can unlock newfound vitality, energy, and resilience.

CHAPTER 14: HORMONAL IMBALANCE

Hormonal imbalance refers to disruptions in the normal levels or activity of hormones in the body, which can have wide-ranging effects on various physiological processes and systems.

Hormones are chemical messengers produced by endocrine glands and other tissues in the body, and they play crucial roles in regulating growth, metabolism, reproduction, mood, sleep, and other functions.

Let's address hormones, their functions, factors contributing to hormonal imbalance, and strategies for maintaining balance. These signaling molecules travel through the bloodstream to target cells or tissues, where they initiate cellular responses.

Hormones regulate a wide range of physiological processes, including:

- Growth and development
- Metabolism and energy balance
- Reproduction and sexual function
- Mood and emotional regulation
- Sleep-wake cycles

- Stress response and adaptation
- Immune function
- Fluid and electrolyte balance
- Blood pressure regulation
- Bone health and calcium metabolism
- Body temperature regulation

Hormones are produced by specialized glands known as endocrine glands, including:

- Pituitary gland
- Thyroid gland
- Adrenal glands
- Pancreas
- Gonads (testes in males, ovaries in females)
- Pineal gland
- Parathyroid glands

Chronic stress and traumatic experiences can disrupt the normal functioning of the hypothalamic-pituitary-adrenal axis, a key regulatory system involved in the stress response. This can lead to dysregulation of cortisol, the body's primary stress hormone, as well as other hormones such as adrenaline and noradrenaline, contributing to hormonal imbalance.

As we age, cellular function and enzyme activity may decline, leading to decreased hormone production, altered hormone metabolism, and impaired hormonal signaling. This can contribute to hormonal imbalances commonly observed in middle-aged and older adults, such as declining levels of sex hormones (e.g., estrogen, testosterone) and changes in insulin sensitivity.

Enzymes play crucial roles in hormone synthesis, metabolism, and signaling pathways. Reduced enzyme activity or impaired enzymatic function can disrupt hormone production and metabolism, contributing to imbalances. For example, deficiencies in enzymes involved in steroid hormone synthesis or metabolism can lead to imbalances in sex hormones.

Exposure to heavy metals, such as lead, mercury, cadmium, and arsenic, can interfere with hormone production and signaling pathways. Heavy metals can disrupt hormone receptors, interfere with hormone synthesis and secretion, and impair hormone metabolism and clearance from the body.

Emerging evidence suggests that exposure to microplastics, tiny plastic particles found in the environment and food chain, may disrupt endocrine function and contribute to hormonal imbalances. Microplastics can act as endocrine-disrupting chemicals, interfering with hormone production, receptor signaling, and metabolism.

Genetic mutations or deletions affecting genes involved in hormone synthesis, metabolism, or signaling pathways can predispose individuals to hormonal imbalances and endocrine disorders. For example, mutations in genes encoding enzymes involved in steroid hormone synthesis can lead to congenital adrenal hyperplasia or other endocrine disorders.

Excess estrogen levels, whether due to endogenous factors (e.g., obesity, hormone therapy) or exogenous sources (e.g., hormone-disrupting chemicals, estrogenic medications), can disrupt hormonal balance and increase the risk of estrogen-related conditions, such as breast endometrial cancer, or prostate cancers.

△△△

Maintaining hormonal balance is key. Consuming a balanced diet rich in fruits, vegetables, whole grains, lean proteins, healthy fats, and fiber can support this. Certain foods, such as cantaloupe, plums, apples, cherries, and pomegranates, contain phytochemicals and antioxidants that may help regulate hormone levels.

Certain supplements, such as omega-3 fatty acids, vitamin D, magnesium, zinc, and adaptogenic herbs (e.g., ashwagandha, Rhodiola), can support hormonal balance and stress resilience.

Maintaining a healthy lifestyle, including regular physical activity, adequate sleep, stress management techniques (e.g., meditation, yoga), and minimizing exposure to environmental toxins (e.g., heavy metals, endocrine-disrupting chemicals), can help support hormonal balance and overall well-being.

There are medications to address hormone-related conditions. Hormone replacement therapy (HRT), oral contraceptives, thyroid hormone replacement, insulin therapy, and other Rx options may be used under the guidance of a healthcare provider to restore hormonal balance and manage hormonal disorders.

Hormonal balance is essential for overall health and well-being. Disruptions in hormone levels or activity can affect various physiological processes. This may include stress, aging, environmental toxins, genetic factors, and lifestyle factors.

Here are the most common hormonal disorders or diseases affecting both men and women, followed by holistic and allopathic approaches for addressing each:

- Hypothyroidism occurs when the thyroid gland does not produce enough thyroid hormones, leading to fatigue, weight gain, cold intolerance, constipation, and hair.

- Hyperthyroidism is characterized by an overactive thyroid gland that produces excess thyroid hormones, causing symptoms such as weight loss, rapid heartbeat, heat intolerance, tremors, and anxiety.

- Polycystic Ovary Syndrome (PCOS) is a hormonal disorder that affects women of reproductive age and is characterized by irregular menstrual periods, excess androgen levels, ovarian cysts, and symptoms such as acne, hirsutism (excessive hair growth), and infertility.

- Type 2 diabetes is a metabolic disorder characterized by insulin resistance and high blood sugar levels. Hormonal imbalances involving insulin, glucagon, and other hormones contribute to impaired glucose metabolism and the development of diabetes.

- Disorders of the adrenal glands, such as adrenal insufficiency (Addison's disease) and Cushing's syndrome, can disrupt hormone production and secretion, leading to symptoms such as fatigue, weakness, weight changes, and alterations in blood pressure and electrolyte levels.

- Menopause is a natural transition in women, typically occurring in their late 40s to early 50s, marked by the cessation of menstrual periods and declining levels of estrogen and progesterone. Hormonal changes during menopause can cause symptoms such as hot flashes, night sweats, mood swings, and vaginal dryness.

Holistic approaches include:

- Adopting a balanced diet rich in whole foods, fiber, lean proteins, healthy fats, and low-glycemic carbohydrates can support hormonal balance and metabolic health. Avoiding processed foods, excessive sugar, and refined carbohydrates can help regulate blood sugar and insulin levels.

- Practicing stress-reducing techniques such as meditation, yoga, deep breathing exercises, and mindfulness can help regulate cortisol levels and support adrenal health. Prioritizing adequate sleep, regular physical activity, and relaxation can also mitigate the impact of stress on hormonal balance.

- Regular exercise, including aerobic exercise, strength training, and flexibility exercises, can improve insulin sensitivity, promote weight management, and support overall hormonal balance. Aim for at least 150 minutes of moderate-intensity exercise per week, along with strength training exercises at least twice a week.

- Certain herbs and botanicals have been traditionally used to support hormonal health and address specific hormonal imbalances. Examples include chasteberry (Vitex agnus-castus) for menstrual irregularities, ashwagandha (Withania somnifera) for stress support, and saw palmetto (Serenoa repens) for prostate health in men.

- Nutritional supplements such as omega-3 fatty acids, vitamin D, magnesium, chromium, and adaptogenic herbs (e.g., Rhodiola, holy basil) may support hormonal balance and metabolic health.

Consult with a healthcare provider before starting any new supplement regimen, especially if you have underlying health conditions or are taking medications.

Allopathic approaches include:

- Depending on the specific hormonal disorder or disease, medications may be prescribed to regulate hormone levels, manage symptoms, and address underlying causes. Examples include thyroid hormone replacement therapy for hypothyroidism, anti-thyroid medications or radioactive iodine therapy for hyperthyroidism, oral contraceptives or anti-androgen medications for PCOS, insulin therapy for diabetes, and hormone replacement therapy (HRT) for menopausal symptoms.

- In some cases, surgical interventions may be necessary to treat hormonal disorders or diseases. For example, surgical removal of the thyroid gland (thyroidectomy) may be recommended for hyperthyroidism or thyroid cancer. At the same time, ovarian drilling or ovarian cystectomy may be performed for PCOS-related infertility or ovarian cysts.

- Allopathic approaches often emphasize lifestyle modifications such as dietary changes, weight management, smoking cessation, and regular physical activity to optimize hormonal health and improve overall well-being.

- For complex hormonal disorders or diseases, consultation with an endocrinologist, a healthcare provider specializing in hormones and the endocrine system, may be warranted.

Endocrinologists can provide comprehensive evaluation, diagnosis, and management of hormonal imbalances using a combination of medical, surgical, and lifestyle interventions.

Integrating lifestyle modifications, dietary changes, stress management techniques, herbal remedies, supplements, medications, and surgical interventions as appropriate can help restore hormonal balance, alleviate symptoms, and improve overall health and well-being.

ΔΔΔ

Sleep plays a crucial role in maintaining overall health and well-being, including hormonal balance. During sleep, the body undergoes various physiological processes that help regulate hormone levels and support various bodily functions.

Several key hormones involved in various bodily functions are influenced by sleep, including:

- Growth hormone: Secreted primarily during deep sleep stages, growth hormone plays a crucial role in tissue repair, muscle growth, and overall growth and development.

- Cortisol: Often referred to as the "stress hormone," cortisol levels typically decrease during sleep, with levels peaking in the early morning hours to help regulate the sleep-wake cycle and prepare the body for the day ahead.

- Leptin and ghrelin: These hormones regulate appetite and hunger signals. Sleep deprivation can disrupt the balance of these hormones, leading to increased hunger and appetite, which may contribute to weight gain and obesity.

- Insulin: Sleep deprivation can also affect insulin sensitivity and glucose metabolism, increasing the risk of insulin resistance and type 2 diabetes.

Chronic sleep deprivation or poor sleep quality can disrupt the body's hormonal balance, leading to a variety of adverse health effects:

- Increased cortisol levels: Sleep deprivation can lead to elevated cortisol levels, which may contribute to stress, inflammation, and metabolic dysfunction.

- appetite regulation: Sleep loss can disrupt the balance of leptin and ghrelin, leading to increased appetite, cravings for high-calorie foods, and weight gain.

- Impaired glucose metabolism: Sleep deprivation is associated with insulin resistance, impaired glucose tolerance, and an increased risk of type 2 diabetes.

- Decreased growth hormone secretion: Inadequate sleep can impair growth hormone secretion, potentially affecting tissue repair, muscle growth, and overall growth and development.

CHAPTER 15: ANXIETY & THE MAGNESIUM FIX

Anxiety is a complex and multifaceted mental health condition that affects millions of individuals worldwide. From the subtle ping of nervousness before a presentation to debilitating panic attacks, anxiety manifests in various forms and intensities, impacting both mental and physical well-being.

Let's examine anxiety, exploring its causes, genetic factors, physiological impacts, and potential overlaps with other health conditions. We'll also explore the role of magnesium in anxiety management, including tests to measure magnesium levels, organs and hormones involved in magnesium regulation, and strategies for supplementation through both dietary sources and supplements.

Anxiety can stem from a combination of genetic, environmental, and psychological factors, making it a complex condition with diverse triggers. Some common causes of anxiety include:

- Genetic predisposition: Certain genetic factors may increase susceptibility to anxiety disorders, though the precise genes involved are still being researched.

- Traumatic experiences: Past trauma or stressful life events, such as abuse, accidents, or loss, can contribute to the development of anxiety disorders.

- Brain chemistry: Imbalances in neurotransmitters like serotonin, dopamine, and norepinephrine may play a role in anxiety by affecting mood regulation and stress response.

- Environmental stressors: Chronic stress, financial problems, work pressure, relationship issues, and major life changes can exacerbate anxiety symptoms.

- Medical conditions: Certain medical conditions, including thyroid disorders, heart disease, respiratory disorders, and chronic pain conditions, may coexist with anxiety or exacerbate its symptoms.

Several gene groups and specific genes have been implicated in predisposing individuals to anxiety disorders. These include:

- Serotonin transporter gene (SLC6A4): Variations in the SLC6A4 gene, which encodes the serotonin transporter protein, have been associated with increased susceptibility to anxiety disorders.

- COMT gene: The catechol-O-methyltransferase (COMT) gene regulates the breakdown of neurotransmitters like dopamine and norepinephrine, and certain variants have been linked to heightened anxiety.

- BDNF gene: Brain-derived neurotrophic factor (BDNF) is involved in neuronal growth and plasticity, and alterations in the BDNF gene have been implicated in anxiety and mood disorders.

- GABA receptor genes: Gamma-aminobutyric acid (GABA) is an inhibitory neurotransmitter that helps regulate anxiety, and variations in genes encoding GABA receptors have been associated with anxiety disorders.

Anxiety doesn't just affect the mind—it can have profound effects on the body as well. Chronic anxiety can lead to:

- Increased heart rate and blood pressure: Anxiety triggers the body's "fight or flight" response, leading to physiological changes like elevated heart rate and blood pressure, which can increase the risk of cardiovascular problems.

- Muscle tension and pain: Persistent anxiety can cause muscle tension, leading to headaches, back pain, jaw pain, and other physical discomforts.

- Digestive issues: Anxiety can disrupt digestion and lead to symptoms like stomach cramps, diarrhea, constipation, and irritable bowel syndrome (IBS).

- Weakened immune function: Prolonged stress and anxiety can suppress the immune system, making individuals more susceptible to infections and illnesses.

- Sleep disturbances: Anxiety often disrupts sleep patterns, leading to insomnia, frequent awakenings, and non-restorative sleep, which can further exacerbate anxiety symptoms.

Anxiety symptoms can sometimes mimic those of heart problems, leading to confusion and misdiagnosis. Common symptoms shared by anxiety and heart issues include:

- Chest pain or discomfort: Both anxiety attacks and heart attacks can cause chest pain or discomfort, though the nature of the pain may differ.
- Shortness of breath: Anxiety-induced hyperventilation can result in shortness of breath, as it can cause certain heart conditions like heart failure or arrhythmias.
- Palpitations: Anxiety can cause rapid or irregular heartbeats (palpitations), similar to those experienced during cardiac arrhythmias.
- Dizziness or lightheadedness: Both anxiety and heart issues can cause feelings of dizziness or lightheadedness, though the underlying mechanisms may vary.

Magnesium plays a crucial role in regulating neurotransmitter function, muscle contraction, and stress response, making it relevant to anxiety management. Tests to measure magnesium levels in the body include:

- Serum magnesium test: This blood test measures the concentration of magnesium in the bloodstream and is commonly used to assess overall magnesium status.
- Red blood cell (RBC) magnesium test: RBC magnesium levels may more accurately reflect

intracellular magnesium status than serum levels.

- Magnesium loading test: In this test, individuals are given a dose of magnesium, and urine samples are collected to assess urinary magnesium excretion, providing insights into magnesium absorption and retention.

Several organs and hormones play key roles in magnesium regulation within the body, including:

- Kidneys: The kidneys help maintain magnesium balance by adjusting urinary excretion based on dietary intake and body needs.

- Parathyroid hormone (PTH): PTH stimulates the release of magnesium from bone stores and enhances renal reabsorption of magnesium to maintain serum levels.

- Vitamin D: Vitamin D facilitates intestinal absorption of magnesium by upregulating the expression of magnesium transport channels in the intestine.

- Thyroid hormones: Thyroid hormones influence magnesium metabolism and transport, with hypothyroidism associated with decreased magnesium levels.

To support magnesium levels and alleviate anxiety symptoms, consider incorporating the following strategies:

- Dietary sources: Consume magnesium-rich foods such as leafy greens (spinach, kale), nuts and seeds (almonds, pumpkin seeds), legumes (beans, lentils), whole grains (quinoa, brown rice), and seafood (salmon, mackerel).

- Supplements: Consider magnesium supplements in various forms, including magnesium citrate, magnesium glycinate, magnesium oxide, or magnesium threonate, under the guidance of a healthcare provider.

- Epsom salt baths: Soaking in Epsom salt baths allows for transdermal absorption of magnesium through the skin, promoting relaxation and muscle tension relief.

- Transdermal magnesium oil: Applying magnesium oil topically allows for absorption through the skin, bypassing the digestive system and potentially minimizing gastrointestinal side effects.

- Magnesium-rich herbs: Incorporate herbs like passionflower, chamomile, and valerian root, which contain magnesium and have calming properties that can help reduce anxiety symptoms.

- Balanced supplementation: Opt for balanced magnesium supplementation with complementary nutrients like calcium, vitamin D, and vitamin K to maintain optimal mineral balance and absorption.

Different forms of magnesium offer unique benefits and absorption rates, allowing for tailored supplementation based on individual needs and preferences.

Here's a list of various forms of magnesium supplements available:

- Magnesium citrate: This form is one of the most used due to its high bioavailability and effectiveness. It's well-absorbed by the body and often used for constipation relief and muscle relaxation.

- Magnesium glycinate: Known for its high absorption rate and gentle effect on the digestive system, magnesium glycinate is popular among those with sensitive stomachs. It's less likely to cause diarrhea compared to other forms.

- Magnesium oxide: While magnesium oxide has a higher magnesium content, it's not as readily absorbed by the body. It's often used as a laxative and to relieve acid indigestion.

- Magnesium sulfate (Epsom salt): Typically used in baths for transdermal absorption through the skin, Epsom salt baths are believed to promote relaxation, ease muscle soreness, and improve sleep quality.

- Magnesium chloride: This form of magnesium is known for its high absorption rate and bioavailability. It's often used in topical magnesium oil or spray for transdermal absorption.

- Magnesium threonate: Known for its ability to cross the blood-brain barrier, magnesium threonate may support cognitive function and brain health. It's often used as a supplement to promote mental clarity and focus.

- Magnesium orotate: This form of magnesium is bound to orotic acid, which is believed to enhance its bioavailability. It's often used to support heart health and may positively affect cardiovascular function.

- Magnesium taurate: A combination of magnesium with the amino acid taurine, magnesium taurate is believed to support cardiovascular health and promote relaxation without causing drowsiness.

- Magnesium malate: This form of magnesium is bound to malic acid, which is involved in energy production within cells. It's often used to support muscle function, reduce fatigue, and alleviate symptoms of fibromyalgia.

- Magnesium carbonate: While less common as a supplement, magnesium carbonate is sometimes used as an antacid to relieve heartburn and acid indigestion. It's also used in some laxative formulations.

It's important to note that the effectiveness and absorption rates of magnesium supplements can vary depending on individual factors such as overall health, digestive function, and existing deficiencies.

CHAPTER 16: CANCER A.K.A. SEVERE OXIDATIVE STRESS

There has been a trend of increasing cancer incidence rates in the U.S., partly due to factors such as aging populations, lifestyle changes, environmental exposures, and advancements in cancer detection and screening methods.

As a result, there is a growing need for more comprehensive genetic testing for cancer to understand individual cancer risks better, guide personalized treatment decisions, and improve outcomes for cancer patients.

"Cancer" is a complex and multifaceted disease characterized by uncontrolled cell growth and proliferation. The actual word "cancer" is a marketing term owned by the pharmaceutical industry.

In scientific terminology, cancer can simply be understood as severe oxidative stress.

This is caused by faulty or deleted genes, inflammation of the digestive system and accessory organs, buildup of toxic cell debris and overgrowth of harmful free radicals, hormonal imbalance from mineral deficiency, and septic blood that goes uncleaned by the liver and is recirculated throughout the body.

The top cancers in America vary depending on age, sex, and geographic location. However, some of the most common U.S. cancers include:

- Breast Cancer: Among women, breast cancer is the most diagnosed cancer and the second leading cause of cancer-related deaths.

- Lung Cancer: Lung cancer is the leading cause of cancer-related deaths in both men and women, primarily due to smoking and exposure to environmental toxins such as radon and asbestos.

- Prostate Cancer: Prostate cancer is the most common cancer diagnosed in men, excluding skin cancer. Although it has a high survival rate when detected early, it remains a significant health concern.

- Colorectal Cancer: Colorectal cancer affects both men and women and is the third most common cancer diagnosed in the United States. Screening and early detection can significantly improve outcomes for colorectal cancer patients.

- Skin Cancer: Skin cancer, including melanoma and non-melanoma skin cancers, is among the most common cancers diagnosed in the United States, with increasing incidence rates in recent years.

- Bladder Cancer: Bladder cancer is more common in men than in women and is often linked to smoking and exposure to certain chemicals.

- Non-Hodgkin Lymphoma: Non-Hodgkin lymphoma is a type of cancer that affects the lymphatic system and can occur at any age, with increasing incidence rates in recent years.

- Kidney Cancer: Kidney cancer, including renal cell carcinoma, is among the top ten most common cancers diagnosed in the United States, with higher incidence rates in men than in women.

- Thyroid Cancer: Thyroid cancer incidence rates have been increasing steadily in recent years, although it remains relatively rare compared to other cancers.

- Leukemia: Leukemia is a cancer of the blood and bone marrow and can affect people of all ages, with different subtypes having varying prognoses and treatment approaches.

Several factors can contribute to severe oxidative stress, including:

- Environmental toxins and pollutants
- Chronic inflammation
- Poor diet high in processed foods, sugar, and unhealthy fats
- Smoking and tobacco use
- Radiation exposure
- Mitochondrial dysfunction
- Liver disease
- Genetic mutations and deletions

ΔΔΔ

One key gene group involved in oxidative stress and

detoxification is the Glutathione S-transferase (GST) family, specifically the GSTM1 gene. This gene encodes an enzyme that plays a crucial role in the detoxification of cancer-causing compounds by conjugating them with glutathione, a powerful antioxidant naturally produced by the body.

Individuals with a deletion or mutation in the GSTM1 gene may have reduced or impaired detoxification capacity due to reduced or nonexistent glutathione production. This will lead to increased accumulation of carcinogens and other harmful compounds, which can contribute to the development of cancer and other oxidative stress-related diseases.

Individuals with a functional GSTM1 gene have a more efficient detoxification capacity. Those with a deletion or mutation in the GSTM1 gene may have impaired detoxification and increased susceptibility to oxidative stress and carcinogen exposure.

ΔΔΔ

Holistic therapies for severe oxidative stress focus on supporting the body's natural detoxification pathways, promoting liver health, enhancing antioxidant defenses, and alkalizing the body and blood.

Key strategies include:

- Liver Cleansing: Incorporating liver-supportive herbs and nutrients such as milk thistle, dandelion root, turmeric, and artichoke can help promote liver detoxification and reduce oxidative stress.
- Blood Cleansing: Herbs like burdock root, red clover, and cleavers can support blood cleansing

and the removal of toxins and impurities from the bloodstream. Additionally, supplementing with glutathione, a powerful antioxidant produced naturally in the body, can enhance blood cleansing and support overall detoxification. Glutathione can be obtained through nutrition from sulfur-rich foods such as garlic, onions, cruciferous vegetables, and avocados. However, liquid glutathione is considered the best method for supplementation as it has high bioavailability and can effectively replenish glutathione levels in the body.

- Arterial Health: Nitric oxide precursors like L-arginine and L-citrulline can support arterial function and blood flow, while nutrients like coenzyme Q10 (CoQ10) and resveratrol can help reduce plaque buildup in the arteries and protect against oxidative damage. Resveratrol, a polyphenol found in red grapes, berries, and peanuts, has antioxidant and anti-inflammatory properties that support cardiovascular health and may help prevent the progression of atherosclerosis by reducing inflammation and improving endothelial function.

- Blood Cell Health: Nutrients such as folate, vitamin B12, and iron are essential for red blood cell production and function, while antioxidants like vitamins C and E can help protect blood cells from oxidative stress and damage. Additionally, resveratrol supplementation can support blood cell health by enhancing antioxidant defenses and improving circulation, thereby promoting overall cardiovascular health and reducing the risk of oxidative damage to blood cells.

- Alkalizing the Body and Blood: Alkalizing the body and blood can help counteract acidity and reduce oxidative stress. Strategies for alkalizing include juicing with alkaline-rich fruits and vegetables such as kale, spinach, cucumber, lemon, and celery. High-antioxidant fruits like berries, cherries, and pomegranates can also support alkalinity and provide hydration. Additionally, consuming high-pH water and fruit-infused water can help alkalinize the body and promote cellular hydration. Fruit contains the converted form of water, $H3O2$, which has smaller water molecules that can penetrate cells more readily, oxygenating and hydrating them effectively.

Allopathic solutions to cancer typically include conventional treatments such as surgery, chemotherapy, radiation therapy, targeted therapy, and immunotherapy. These treatments aim to target and destroy cancer cells directly or inhibit their growth and spread.

While these approaches can be effective in treating cancer and improving survival rates, they often do not fully address the underlying factors contributing to cancer development or support the body's detox organs, systems, and cellular-level functionality.

These treatments do not typically prioritize the restoration of essential vitamins and minerals that may become depleted during cancer treatment or because of the disease itself.

As a result, there may be missed opportunities to optimize the body's natural defenses and support overall health during and after cancer treatment.

Integrative approaches that combine conventional cancer treatments with complementary therapies focused on detoxification, nutritional support, and overall wellness may offer a more comprehensive care.

△△△

Allopathic genetic testing for cancer typically involves analyzing specific genetic mutations or alterations known to be associated with certain types of cancer. These tests may include testing for mutations in genes such as BRCA1 and BRCA2 for breast and ovarian cancer, KRAS and EGFR for lung cancer, and APC and TP53 for colorectal cancer.

These tests are often used to assess an individual's risk of developing cancer, guide treatment decisions, and inform personalized treatment approaches.

However, it's important to note that allopathic diagnostic genetic testing for cancer may not typically include testing for key gene groups related to methylation, inflammation response, detoxification, lipid metabolism, bone density, oxidative stress, or insulin sensitivity.

These gene groups play important roles in how cancer can develop and progress, but they are not routinely assessed as part of standard genetic testing protocols in allopathic medicine.

Expanded genetic testing may provide insights into a broader range of genetic factors impacting overall health and disease risk, including genes related to detoxification pathways, inflammation regulation, hormonal balance, and nutrient metabolism.

By enhancing medical education in these areas, healthcare providers can better meet the evolving needs of cancer patients and improve overall cancer prevention, diagnosis, and treatment outcomes.

CHAPTER 17: THE GUT-BRAIN AXIS

The gut-brain axis plays a significant role in the development and progression of various diseases and disorders, with numerous conditions being influenced by the communication between the gut and the brain.

Some of the diseases and disorders related to the gut-brain axis include:

- Irritable Bowel Syndrome (IBS)
- Inflammatory Bowel Disease (IBD), including Crohn's disease and ulcerative colitis
- Gastroesophageal Reflux Disease (GERD)
- Functional Dyspepsia
- Gastroparesis
- Celiac disease
- Non-Celiac Gluten Sensitivity
- Small Intestinal Bacterial Overgrowth (SIBO)
- Food intolerances and allergies
- Eating disorders, such as anorexia nervosa and bulimia nervosa
- Anxiety disorders, including generalized anxiety disorder and panic disorder
- Depression
- Autism Spectrum Disorder (ASD)

- Attention Deficit Hyperactivity Disorder (ADHD)
- Migraine headaches
- Neurodegenerative diseases, such as Parkinson's disease and Alzheimer's disease
- Mood disorders, including bipolar disorder

The prevalence of gut-brain axis-related diseases and disorders has been seen in recent years, with increasing recognition of the importance of gut microbiota and its influence on brain health. Factors such as changes in diet, lifestyle, and environmental exposures have contributed to the increasing incidence and prevalence of these conditions.

Other reasons for this include rising levels of chronic stress, fatigue and aging populations. Understanding and addressing the interplay between the gut and the brain is essential for preventing and managing gut-brain many diseases and disorders in the future.

The gut-brain axis refers to the communication system between the gastrointestinal tract (the gut) and the brain. This connection is crucial for regulating various physiological processes and plays a significant role in overall health and well-being.

The gut-brain axis is essential for maintaining homeostasis and regulating mood, cognition, immune function, and even behavior. The two systems communicate through neural, hormonal, and immune pathways, influencing each other's function and activity.

The gut, or gastrointestinal tract, is responsible for the digestion and absorption of nutrients and houses trillions of microorganisms collectively known as the gut microbiota. This microbiota plays a key role in nutrient metabolism, immune regulation, and neurotransmitter production.

The brain, as the central nervous system, coordinates various bodily functions, including perception, cognition, emotion, and behavior. It receives signals from the gut via the vagus nerve and other neural pathways, influencing mood, appetite, and stress responses.

The gut produces neurotransmitters, such as serotonin, dopamine, and gamma-aminobutyric acid (GABA), which the brain utilizes to regulate mood and behavior. Conversely, the brain can influence gut function through the release of stress hormones and neurotransmitters, impacting gastrointestinal motility, secretion, and immune function.

NEUROTRANSMITTERS & THEIR FUNCTIONS

- Serotonin: Regulates mood, appetite, and sleep.
- Dopamine: Involved in reward and motivation, motor control, and mood regulation.
- Gamma-aminobutyric acid (GABA): Inhibitory neurotransmitter that reduces neuronal excitability, promoting relaxation and reducing anxiety.
- Acetylcholine: Plays a role in learning, memory, and muscle contraction.
- Norepinephrine: Involved in the body's "fight or flight" response and arousal.
- Glutamate: Major excitatory neurotransmitter involved in learning and memory.
- Histamine: Regulates sleep-wake cycles, appetite, and immune responses.
- Endorphins: Natural painkillers produced in response to stress or pain.
- Oxytocin: Regulates social bonding, trust, and empathy.

- Cortisol: Stress hormone involved in the body's stress response and regulation of metabolism.

The gut-brain axis is a complex, bidirectional communication system that plays a vital role in regulating various physiological processes and maintaining gut and brain health. The brain is divided into several main parts, each with its own functions and responsibilities:

- Cerebrum: The largest part of the brain, consisting of two hemispheres (left and right). The cerebrum is responsible for higher cognitive functions such as thinking, memory, perception, and voluntary movement.

- Cerebellum: Located beneath the cerebrum at the back of the brain, the cerebellum coordinates voluntary movements, balance, and posture. It also plays a role in motor learning and cognitive functions.

- Brainstem: Situated at the base of the brain, the brainstem connects the brain to the spinal cord and controls basic bodily functions such as heart rate, breathing, and swallowing. It consists of the midbrain, pons, and medulla oblongata.

- Diencephalon: Located between the cerebrum and the brainstem, the diencephalon includes structures such as the thalamus and hypothalamus. The thalamus relays sensory information to the cerebral cortex, while the hypothalamus regulates hormone secretion, body temperature, thirst, hunger, and sleep.

This bidirectional communication system links the central nervous system (CNS) to the enteric nervous system (ENS) in the gastrointestinal tract through the following pathways:

- Neural Pathways: The vagus nerve serves as a major conduit for communication between the gut and the brain, transmitting signals bidirectionally. Sensory information from the gut travels to the brain, influencing mood, cognition, and behavior, while motor signals from the brain modulate gastrointestinal motility, secretion, and immune function.

- Hormonal Pathways: The gut produces and releases various hormones and neuropeptides that can influence brain function and behavior. For example, serotonin, a neurotransmitter primarily produced in the gut, plays a key role in mood regulation and is implicated in conditions such as depression and anxiety.

- Immune Pathways: The gut is home to a vast array of immune cells and microbiota that interact with the immune system and produce cytokines and other signaling molecules. Dysregulation of the gut microbiota can lead to inflammation, which has been implicated in various brain disorders, including depression, autism, and neurodegenerative diseases.

The brain can influence gut function through the release of stress hormones and neurotransmitters, impacting gastrointestinal motility, secretion, and immune function. This bidirectional communication between the brain and the gut is essential for maintaining homeostasis, regulating mood, cognition, immune function, and behavior, and supporting overall health and well-being.

Detoxifying the gut-brain axis involves supporting gut health through a balanced diet, adequate hydration, probiotics, and prebiotics to maintain a healthy gut microbiota. Additionally, reducing exposure to environmental toxins, managing stress, and promoting relaxation techniques can help support the optimal functioning of the gut-brain axis.

Nutrient-rich foods, such as fruits, vegetables, whole grains, lean proteins, and healthy fats, support brain and gut health. Supplements like omega-3 fatty acids, probiotics, digestive enzymes, and vitamins and minerals (e.g., B vitamins and magnesium) can also enhance gut function and support brain health.

Allopathic treatments for gut and brain disorders may include medications, such as proton pump inhibitors for gastrointestinal issues and antidepressants or anxiolytics for mood disorders. However, these treatments may not address underlying imbalances in the gut microbiota or nutritional deficiencies.

Chiropractic care can help support the gut-brain axis by addressing spinal misalignments (subluxations) that may interfere with nervous system function. By restoring proper spinal alignment and nerve function, chiropractic adjustments can promote optimal communication between the gut and brain.

Genetic testing for brain health can identify mutations or deletions within the genetic code that may impact neurotransmitter production or metabolism. Understanding genetic predispositions can help tailor treatment approaches and support optimal brain function.

CHAPTER 18: DERMAL DETOX

Skin, the largest organ of the human body, serves as a protective barrier against environmental toxins, pathogens, and physical damage. However, its complex structure and susceptibility to various internal and external factors make it prone to a myriad of issues, ranging from minor irritations to chronic conditions with profound impacts on physical and emotional well-being.

Skin forms through cell differentiation and maturation, with various layers contributing to its structure. Repair involves cell proliferation and migration to replace damaged tissue, accompanied by inflammation.

The skin consists of three main layers: the epidermis, dermis, and subcutaneous tissue, each with distinct roles in maintaining its integrity and function. The epidermis, the outermost layer, serves as a protective barrier, while the dermis provides structural support and houses essential structures like blood vessels and hair follicles. Beneath these layers lies the subcutaneous tissue, which contains fat cells and provides insulation and cushioning for the body.

Skin diseases encompass a wide range of conditions that affect the skin's health and appearance, from common issues like acne and eczema to more serious conditions such as psoriasis and skin cancer. Controversial conditions like Morgellons disease add complexity to the landscape of dermatological concerns.

Understanding the causes and mechanisms behind these skin diseases involves delving into the intricate interplay of genetic factors, immune responses, environmental influences, and cellular processes.

We'll explore the top skin diseases, delve into the gene groups responsible for skin health, discuss how skin is formed and repaired, and provide insights into holistic and allopathic approaches for addressing these conditions effectively.

An unbalanced gut, compounded by advanced Candida and/or parasitic infections, can profoundly impact skin health and contribute to a myriad of dermatological issues.

When the delicate equilibrium of the gut microbiome is disrupted, opportunistic pathogens like Candida albicans or parasites can proliferate, leading to systemic inflammation and immune dysregulation.

Candida overgrowth, often fueled by factors such as poor diet, stress, or prolonged antibiotic use, can compromise intestinal integrity and promote the release of toxins into the bloodstream, triggering inflammatory responses throughout the body.

Additionally, parasitic infections may further disrupt gut function and exacerbate nutrient deficiencies, impairing the body's ability to maintain healthy skin.

And, genetic mutations or deletions within skin gene groups

can heighten susceptibility to skin disorders, as impaired collagen production, compromised skin barrier function, and dysregulated immune responses create fertile ground for conditions like acne, eczema, psoriasis, and dermatitis to arise and persist.

Addressing gut dysbiosis, combating Candida and parasitic infections, and addressing genetic predispositions are crucial components of comprehensive strategies for effectively managing and resolving skin issues.

Skin diseases encompass a broad spectrum of conditions, ranging from benign to severe, each with unique characteristics and triggers.

Among the most prevalent skin issues are:

- Acne: Caused by excess oil production, clogged pores, bacteria, and inflammation.
- Eczema: An inflammatory skin condition characterized by dry, itchy, and inflamed skin.
- Psoriasis: A chronic autoimmune disease that leads to the rapid growth of skin cells, resulting in thick, red, and scaly patches.
- Dermatitis: Skin inflammation triggered by irritants, allergens, or genetic factors.
- Skin Cancer: Caused by exposure to ultraviolet (UV) radiation from the sun or artificial sources.
- Morgellons disease: A controversial condition characterized by fibers or unusual materials embedded in the skin, along with symptoms like itching and skin lesions.

Gene groups responsible for skin health include:

COLLAGEN GENES

- Encodes proteins forming the structural framework of the skin.
- Mutations can lead to connective tissue disorders and skin abnormalities.

INFLAMMATORY GENES

- Regulate the inflammatory response in skin conditions.
- Dysregulation can lead to chronic inflammation and immune dysfunction.

SKIN BARRIER GENES

- Form and maintain the skin barrier, protecting against environmental stressors.
- Mutations can impair barrier function, increasing susceptibility to skin disorders.

IMMUNE SYSTEM GENES

- Critical for defending the skin against pathogens and maintaining immune homeostasis.
- Alterations can lead to autoimmune skin diseases and inflammatory responses.

DETOXIFICATION GENES

- Eliminate toxins from the body, crucial for skin health.
- Dysfunctional genes may contribute to skin diseases by impairing toxin removal.

When diluted properly with carrier oils, essential oil combinations can effectively support skin detoxification and repair, leaving the skin rejuvenated, nourished, and glowing with health. Always perform a patch test before use.

Here are some examples:

- Tea Tree Essential Oil: Known for its antimicrobial properties, tea tree oil helps cleanse the skin of impurities and supports the healing of blemishes and breakouts. It's often diluted with jojoba oil or grapeseed oil, which are lightweight and non-comedogenic, making them suitable for all skin types.

- Lavender Essential Oil: Lavender oil is renowned for its calming and soothing properties, making it ideal for sensitive or irritated skin. It helps reduce inflammation, promotes skin regeneration, and aids in detoxification. When combined with carrier oils like sweet almond oil or coconut oil, it provides hydration and nourishment to the skin.

- Frankincense Essential Oil: Frankincense oil has powerful rejuvenating properties that support skin repair and regeneration. It helps diminish the appearance of scars, fine lines, and wrinkles while also promoting overall skin health. When mixed with carrier oils such as rosehip seed oil or argan oil, it enhances moisturization and boosts the skin's natural radiance.

- Geranium Essential Oil: Geranium oil is beneficial for balancing oil production, reducing inflammation, and improving skin texture. It aids in detoxifying the skin, refining pores, and promoting a clear complexion. Evening primrose oil or apricot kernel oil are excellent carrier oils to blend with geranium oil, providing hydration and enhancing skin elasticity.

- Rosemary Essential Oil: Rosemary oil stimulates circulation, which can help detoxify the skin by improving lymphatic drainage and removing toxins. It has antioxidant properties that protect the skin from environmental damage and promote cell renewal. Olive oil or avocado oil are recommended carrier oils to mix with rosemary oil, offering deep hydration and nourishment to the skin.

Colloidal silver spray and colloidal copper spray are topical solutions containing tiny particles of silver or copper suspended in a liquid. These sprays are often used for their potential antibacterial, antifungal, and skin-conditioning properties.

Here's more information about each:

COLLOIDAL SILVER SPRAY

- Benefits: Colloidal silver is believed to have

antimicrobial properties, which may help combat bacteria, viruses, and fungi on the skin. It is commonly used for wound healing, acne treatment, and as a general skin disinfectant.

- Recommended Usage: Apply colloidal silver spray directly to the affected area of the skin, such as cuts, scrapes, burns, or acne-prone areas. Allow it to air dry or gently pat dry with a clean cloth. Repeat application as needed, typically 2-3 times per day. It can also be used as a general skin toner or refreshing spray.

COLLOIDAL COPPER SPRAY

- Benefits: Colloidal copper is believed to have antioxidant and anti-inflammatory properties, which may help promote skin healing, reduce inflammation, and support collagen production. It is commonly used for its potential anti-aging and skin-conditioning effects.

- Recommended Usage: Apply colloidal copper spray to clean and dry skin as needed. It can be used as a toner, facial mist, or spot treatment for areas of concern. Allow it to air dry or gently pat dry with a clean cloth. For best results, use it regularly as part of your skincare routine, either once or twice daily.

When using colloidal silver or copper sprays, following the manufacturer's instructions and guidelines for safe usage is essential. While these sprays are generally considered safe for topical use, some individuals may experience skin irritation or allergic reactions. Remember: the patch test.

It's also important to note that while colloidal silver and copper may benefit skin health, scientific evidence supporting their effectiveness for specific skin conditions is limited. As such, it's best to use these sprays as part of a comprehensive skincare regimen and consult with a healthcare professional if you have any concerns or questions about their use.

Some other holistic approaches to skin healing include:

- Diet: To nourish your skin from within, embrace a balanced diet abundant in fruits, vegetables, omega-rich fats, and lean proteins. Incorporate skin-loving foods like avocados, nuts, and fatty fish while minimizing processed sugars and inflammatory foods. Additionally, consider incorporating essential oils known for their skin-health benefits, such as lavender, tea tree, and frankincense, which can be diluted and applied topically or diffused for aromatherapy.

- Hydration: Hydrate your skin from the inside out by drinking ample water throughout the day. Proper hydration supports skin elasticity, moisture retention, and overall health. Infuse your hydration routine with topical treatments like magnesium lotion, coconut oil, or aloe vera gel to soothe and moisturize dry or irritated skin.

- Stress Management: Prioritize stress-reducing practices like meditation, yoga, or deep breathing exercises to promote skin health and overall well-being. Chronic stress can exacerbate skin conditions, so incorporating relaxation techniques into your daily routine can help maintain a healthy balance.

- Skincare: Opt for gentle cleansers, moisturizers, and sunscreen to protect and nourish your skin. Consider incorporating natural remedies like castor oil, black seed oil, magnesium lotion, or calendula-infused creams to soothe inflammation, promote healing, and maintain skin integrity. Regular exfoliation with gentle scrubs or chemical exfoliants can also help unclog pores and promote cell turnover.

- Supplements: Enhance your skin's resilience with targeted supplements like omega-3 fatty acids, vitamin D, and probiotics. These nutrients support skin hydration, inflammation regulation, and immune function, contributing to a healthy complexion from the inside out. Additionally, consider incorporating collagen peptides or silica supplements to support skin elasticity and regeneration.

- Lifestyle: Cultivate a healthy lifestyle by exercising regularly, prioritizing restful sleep, and minimizing habits like smoking and excessive alcohol consumption. Physical activity promotes circulation and detoxification, while adequate sleep allows for cellular repair and regeneration. Avoiding tobacco and limiting alcohol intake can help prevent premature aging and maintain skin health in the long run.

Here are some allopathic approaches to skin healing:

- Topical Treatments: Utilized to address localized skin issues, topical treatments encompass a variety of options tailored to specific conditions. Corticosteroids are commonly prescribed to reduce inflammation, itching, and redness associated with conditions like eczema, psoriasis, and dermatitis. Retinoids, derived from vitamin A, promote skin cell turnover, unclog pores, and improve overall skin texture, making them effective in treating acne, fine lines, and hyperpigmentation. Additionally, natural alternatives like tea tree oil, aloe vera gel, and chamomile extract offer soothing and anti-inflammatory properties, making them suitable for sensitive or irritated skin.

- Oral Medications: Oral medications play a pivotal role in managing systemic skin conditions or those resistant to topical treatments. Antibiotics, such as tetracycline or doxycycline, target bacterial infections commonly associated with acne or folliculitis. Antihistamines, like cetirizine or loratadine, alleviate itching and allergic reactions in conditions like urticaria or allergic dermatitis. In severe cases of autoimmune skin diseases like psoriasis or eczema, immunosuppressants like methotrexate or cyclosporine may be prescribed to modulate immune responses and reduce inflammation systemically.

- Phototherapy: Phototherapy, also known as light therapy, harnesses the therapeutic properties of ultraviolet (UV) light to alleviate symptoms of various skin conditions. In conditions like psoriasis, UVB phototherapy slows the growth of affected skin cells and reduces inflammation, leading to improvements in plaque severity and erythema. Narrowband UVB therapy is particularly effective in treating psoriasis lesions, minimizing side effects associated with broader UV exposure. Additionally, UVA phototherapy combined with photosensitizing agents, known as PUVA therapy, is utilized in conditions like vitiligo or cutaneous T-cell lymphoma, targeting abnormal skin cells and promoting repigmentation or cancer cell destruction.

- Surgery: Surgical intervention may be necessary to address certain dermatological concerns, particularly those involving cancerous or abnormal growths. Mohs micrographic surgery, considered the gold standard for treating skin cancer, involves the precise removal of cancerous tissue layers while preserving healthy surrounding skin. Cryotherapy, excisional surgery, and laser surgery are alternative approaches used to remove skin lesions, warts, or benign tumors. Surgical procedures are performed under local anesthesia and may require post-operative wound care and monitoring to ensure optimal healing and cosmetic outcomes.

- Biologic Therapies: Biologic therapies represent a revolutionary approach to treating severe, refractory autoimmune skin diseases by targeting specific molecules involved in the inflammatory cascade. Biologics, derived from living organisms, modulate immune responses and reduce inflammation in conditions like psoriasis, eczema, and hidradenitis suppurativa. Tumor necrosis factor-alpha (TNF-alpha) inhibitors, interleukin-17 (IL-17) inhibitors, and interleukin-23 (IL-23) inhibitors are examples of biologics approved for treating psoriasis, offering rapid and sustained improvements in disease severity and quality of life. These targeted therapies are administered via subcutaneous injections or intravenous infusions and require regular monitoring for safety and efficacy.

Navigating the complex terrain of skin issues requires a

multifaceted approach that addresses underlying causes, triggers, and contributing factors.

CHAPTER 19: WEIGHT LOSS & WEIGHT GAIN

Weight management is a journey filled with challenges, triumphs, setbacks, and successes. It's a topic that captivates millions worldwide, with individuals striving to either shed excess pounds or gain healthy mass.

The path to achieving one's desired weight is not always straightforward, as it involves a multitude of factors ranging from dietary choices and exercise routines to genetics and psychological well-being. We'll explore the both weight loss and weight gain.

Weight loss, often synonymous with phrases like "getting in shape" or "shedding pounds," is a process whereby individuals aim to reduce their body mass through a combination of calorie restriction, increased physical activity, and lifestyle modifications.

At its core, weight loss revolves around the principle of creating a calorie deficit, wherein the calories burned exceed the calories consumed, leading to a decrease in body weight over time.

The journey of weight loss is highly individualized, as factors such as metabolism, body composition, hormonal balance, and genetic predisposition play significant roles.

While crash diets and extreme exercise regimens may yield rapid results, sustainable weight loss is best achieved through gradual, long-term changes that prioritize overall health and well-being.

These changes include adopting a balanced diet rich in fruits, vegetables, lean proteins, and whole grains, along with regular exercise and adequate hydration.

Moreover, understanding the psychological aspects of weight loss is crucial. Many individuals struggle with emotional eating, stress-induced cravings, and negative self-perception, which can hinder progress and lead to cycles of yo-yo dieting.

Building a supportive environment, seeking professional guidance, and cultivating a positive mindset are essential components of a successful weight loss journey.

In the realm of weight loss, myths and misconceptions abound, often perpetuated by fad diets, sensationalized media headlines, and anecdotal success stories.

MYTH #1: CRASH DIETS ARE EFFECTIVE FOR LONG-TERM WEIGHT LOSS

Reality: Crash diets may yield initial results, but they are unsustainable and can lead to nutrient deficiencies, muscle loss, and metabolic damage in the long run.

MYTH #2: CARBOHYDRATES ARE THE ENEMY OF WEIGHT LOSS

Reality: Carbohydrates are a vital source of energy and should be included in a balanced diet. The key is to focus on complex carbohydrates from whole foods like fruits, vegetables, and whole grains while moderating refined sugars and processed foods.

MYTH #3: SPOT REDUCTION EXERCISES TARGET FAT LOSS IN SPECIFIC AREAS

Reality: Spot reduction is a myth; targeted exercises may strengthen and tone specific muscles but do not selectively burn fat in those areas. Overall body fat reduction is achieved through a combination of cardio, strength training, and a calorie-controlled diet.

∆∆∆

While much attention is often given to weight loss, healthy weight gain is equally important, especially for individuals looking to build muscle mass, recover from illness, or overcome undernutrition. Unlike weight loss, which involves a calorie deficit, weight gain requires a calorie surplus, wherein the calories consumed exceed those expended.

To achieve healthy weight gain, focus on nutrient-dense

foods that provide a balance of carbohydrates, proteins, healthy fats, vitamins, and minerals. Incorporate calorie-rich options such as nuts, seeds, avocados, dairy products, lean meats, and whole-grain carbohydrates into your diet. Additionally, prioritize strength training exercises to stimulate muscle growth and enhance overall strength and endurance.

It's essential to approach weight gain with patience and consistency, as rapid increases in body weight can lead to unwanted fat accumulation and metabolic imbalances.

In the realm of weight management, both weight loss and weight gain present unique challenges and opportunities. By understanding the science behind these processes, debunking common myths, and implementing practical strategies, individuals can embark on a journey toward improved health, vitality, and self-confidence.

Sustainable progress takes time, dedication, and a holistic approach that prioritizes both physical and emotional well-being.

Whether your goal is to shed excess pounds or gain healthy mass, embrace the journey, celebrate small victories, and, above all, be kind to yourself along the way.

Here are examples each for ways to lose weight and gain weight holistically and allopathically.

Holistic weight-loss strategies include:

- Mindful Eating: Practice mindful eating by paying attention to hunger and fullness cues, savoring each bite, and avoiding distractions while eating.
- Regular Exercise: Incorporate regular physical activity into your routine, such as brisk walking, jogging, cycling, or yoga, to burn calories and

improve overall fitness.

- **Whole Foods Diet:** Focus on consuming a diet rich in whole, nutrient-dense foods such as fruits, vegetables, lean proteins, whole grains, and healthy fats while minimizing processed and sugary foods.

- **Stress Reduction:** Manage stress through techniques like meditation, deep breathing exercises, yoga, or spending time in nature to reduce emotional eating and cortisol levels.

- **Adequate Sleep:** Prioritize getting enough sleep each night, aiming for 7-9 hours, as inadequate sleep can disrupt hormone balance, increase appetite, and impair metabolism.

- **Hydration:** Drink plenty of water throughout the day, as dehydration can sometimes be mistaken for hunger and lead to overeating.

- **Portion Control:** Practice portion control by using smaller plates, measuring serving sizes, and being mindful of portion sizes to prevent overeating.

- **Intermittent Fasting:** Consider intermittent fasting, which involves cycling between periods of eating and fasting, to promote fat loss and improve metabolic health.

- **Supportive Environment:** Surround yourself with supportive friends, family, or a community to encourage healthy habits and hold you accountable on your weight loss journey.

- **Professional Guidance:** Seek guidance from a registered dietitian, nutritionist, or holistic health practitioner who can provide personalized advice and support tailored to your individual needs and goals.

Allopathic weight-loss strategies include:

- Calorie Restriction: Adopt a calorie-controlled diet that reduces overall calorie intake to create a calorie deficit, leading to weight loss over time.

- Weight Loss Medications: Consider prescription weight loss medications, such as orlistat, phentermine, or liraglutide, under the supervision of a healthcare provider to aid in weight loss.

- Bariatric Surgery: Explore surgical options like gastric bypass, sleeve gastrectomy, or gastric banding for individuals with severe obesity or obesity-related health conditions.

- Medical Meal Replacements: Use medical meal replacement products, such as shakes or bars, prescribed by a healthcare provider to replace meals and support weight loss efforts.

- Appetite Suppressants: Utilize appetite-suppressing medications, such as phentermine or lorcaserin, to reduce hunger and food cravings as part of a comprehensive weight loss plan.

- Weight Loss Programs: Enroll in structured weight loss programs or clinics that offer counseling, meal plans, and behavioral support to help individuals achieve their weight loss goals.

- Monitoring Tools: Use technology tools like fitness trackers, calorie-counting apps, or wearable devices to monitor food intake, physical activity, and weight loss progress.

- Medical Monitoring: Undergo regular medical monitoring and evaluation by a healthcare provider to assess progress, manage any medical conditions, and adjust treatment as needed.

- Behavioral Therapy: Participate in behavioral therapy or counseling sessions with a trained therapist to address emotional eating, binge eating disorder, or other psychological factors contributing to weight gain.

- Lifestyle Modifications: Make lifestyle modifications such as smoking cessation, reducing alcohol intake, and managing underlying medical conditions like diabetes or hypertension to support weight loss efforts and improve overall health.

Holistic weight-gain strategies include:

- Calorie Surplus: Consume a calorie surplus by increasing overall calorie intake to exceed the number of calories burned through metabolism and physical activity.

- Strength Training: Incorporate strength training exercises like weightlifting, resistance bands, or bodyweight exercises to build muscle mass and increase overall body weight.

- Balanced Diet: Eat a balanced diet that includes a variety of nutrient-dense foods, including lean proteins, healthy fats, complex carbohydrates, fruits, vegetables, and dairy products.

- Frequent Meals: Eat frequent, smaller meals throughout the day to increase calorie intake and provide a steady supply of nutrients to support muscle growth and weight gain.

- Nutrient-Rich Snacks: Snack on nutrient-rich foods like nuts, seeds, trail mix, cheese, yogurt, or protein bars between meals to boost calorie intake and support weight gain.

- Healthy Fats: Include healthy fats in your diet from sources like avocados, nuts, seeds, olive oil, and fatty fish to increase calorie density and provide essential nutrients.

- Protein Supplementation: Supplement your diet with protein powders or shakes to increase protein intake and support muscle growth and repair.

- Sleep and Recovery: Ensure adequate sleep and recovery time to allow your body to rest, repair, and build muscle tissue effectively.

- Hydration: Stay hydrated by drinking plenty of fluids throughout the day, including water, milk, fruit juices, and sports drinks, to support overall health and digestion.

- Mindful Eating: Practice mindful eating by paying attention to hunger cues, enjoying your meals, and avoiding distractions to enhance digestion and nutrient absorption.

Allopathic weight-gain strategies include:

- Nutritional Supplements: Use high-calorie nutritional supplements or meal replacement drinks prescribed by a healthcare provider to increase calorie intake and support weight gain.

- Appetite Stimulants: Consider appetite-stimulating medications like megestrol acetate or dronabinol under the guidance of a healthcare provider to increase appetite and food intake.

- Hormone Therapy: Explore hormone replacement therapy or medications like testosterone or growth hormone under medical supervision to address hormonal imbalances contributing to weight loss or muscle wasting.

- Nutrition Counseling: Seek guidance from a registered dietitian or nutritionist who can develop a personalized meal plan tailored to your dietary preferences, calorie needs, and weight gain goals.

- Muscle-building Exercises: Focus on muscle-building exercises and resistance training techniques under the supervision of a fitness professional to promote muscle growth and weight gain.

- Medical Evaluation: Undergo a comprehensive medical evaluation to identify and address any potential underlying medical conditions, digestive disorders, or metabolic issues contributing to weight loss.

- Gastrointestinal Motility Agents: Consider medications like metoclopramide or erythromycin to improve gastrointestinal motility and enhance digestion and absorption of nutrients.

- Enteral Nutrition: In cases of severe malnutrition or inability to eat orally, consider enteral nutrition through feeding tubes or intravenous (IV) nutrition to provide essential nutrients and support weight gain.

- Behavioral Therapy: Participate in behavioral therapy or counseling sessions with a trained therapist to address psychological factors, stressors, or eating disorders that may be affecting appetite and food intake.

- Medical Monitoring: Receive regular medical monitoring and evaluation by a healthcare provider to assess weight gain progress, monitor for any adverse effects or complications, and adjust treatment as needed.

CHAPTER 20: HAIR LOSS & TOOTH LOSS

Hair loss and tooth loss are two common and distressing conditions that can significantly impact an individual's physical appearance, self-esteem, and overall quality of life. While they may seem unrelated, both conditions share underlying causes and consequences that warrant exploration.

Hair loss, medically known as alopecia, refers to the partial or complete loss of hair from the scalp or other parts of the body. It can manifest in various forms, including male-pattern baldness, female-pattern hair loss, alopecia areata, and telogen effluvium.

While hair loss is often associated with aging, it can affect individuals of all ages and genders, with genetics, hormonal imbalances, medical conditions, and lifestyle factors playing significant roles.

One of the primary causes of hair loss is alopecia, a hereditary condition characterized by the gradual thinning of hair follicles due to the influence of hormones such as dihydrotestosterone (DHT).

Other factors contributing to hair loss include stress, poor nutrition, certain medications, autoimmune disorders, and underlying medical conditions like thyroid disorders and alopecia areata.

The psychological impact of hair loss should not be underestimated, as it can lead to feelings of embarrassment, self-consciousness, and diminished self-confidence.

Many individuals experiencing hair loss may seek out treatments and solutions to restore their hairline and regain a sense of normalcy in their appearance.

Let's go through common myths and misconceptions surrounding the condition:

MYTH #1: HAIR LOSS IS SOLELY DETERMINED BY GENETICS

Reality: While genetics play a significant role in hair loss, environmental factors, lifestyle choices, and medical conditions can also contribute to hair thinning and shedding.

MYTH #2: WEARING HATS OR USING HAIR PRODUCTS CAUSES HAIR LOSS

Reality: Wearing hats or using hair products like gel or hairspray does not directly cause hair loss. However, excessive pulling or traction on the hair follicles can lead to a condition known as traction alopecia.

MYTH #3: HAIR LOSS IS IRREVERSIBLE

Reality: While some forms of hair loss may be permanent, many cases can be treated or managed with appropriate medical interventions, lifestyle modifications, and supportive therapies.

ΔΔΔ

Tooth loss an occur due to various factors, including dental decay, gum disease, trauma, congenital abnormalities, and aging. Tooth loss can profoundly affect oral health, speech, chewing function, and facial aesthetics, leading to difficulties in eating, speaking, and smiling confidently.

One of the primary causes of tooth loss is periodontal (gum) disease, a chronic inflammatory condition characterized by the accumulation of plaque and bacteria along the gumline.

If left untreated, gum disease can lead to gum recession, bone loss, and eventual tooth loss. Other factors contributing to tooth loss include dental caries (cavities), trauma from accidents or injuries, poor oral hygiene, smoking, and systemic conditions such as diabetes and osteoporosis.

The consequences of tooth loss extend beyond the oral cavity, impacting overall health and well-being. Individuals with missing teeth may experience nutritional deficiencies, digestive problems, speech impediments, and social stigma associated with dental appearance.

Furthermore, tooth loss can contribute to changes in facial

structure and jaw alignment, leading to bite problems and temporomandibular joint (TMJ) disorders.

Like hair loss, tooth loss is surrounded by myths and misconceptions that can influence perceptions and attitudes toward dental health.

Fortunately, advancements in medical and dental technology have expanded the range of treatment options available for individuals experiencing hair loss and tooth loss.

Hair loss solutions include:

- Topical medications: Minoxidil (Rogaine) and finasteride (Propecia) are FDA-approved medications for treating male and female pattern hair loss by promoting hair growth and preventing further hair loss.
- Oral medications: Finasteride (Propecia) is a prescription medication that inhibits the production of DHT, a hormone implicated in hair loss, thereby promoting hair regrowth and thickening.
- Hair transplantation: Surgical procedures such as follicular unit transplantation (FUT) and follicular unit extraction (FUE) involve harvesting hair follicles from donor areas and transplanting them into balding or thinning areas of the scalp.
- Low-level laser therapy (LLLT): LLLT devices emit non-invasive laser light to stimulate hair follicles, improve blood circulation, and promote hair growth in individuals with androgenetic alopecia.

Tooth loss solutions include:

- Dental implants: Dental implants are titanium posts surgically inserted into the jawbone to replace missing tooth roots. They provide a stable foundation for crowns, bridges, or dentures, restoring chewing function and preventing bone loss.

- Fixed dental bridges: Dental bridges consist of artificial teeth (pontics) anchored to adjacent natural teeth or dental implants, bridging the gap created by missing teeth and restoring dental aesthetics and function.

- Removable dentures: Removable dentures are prosthetic devices designed to replace multiple missing teeth. They can be partial dentures (replacing several teeth) or complete dentures (replacing all teeth) and are custom-made to fit securely in the mouth.

- All-on-4 dental implants: All-on-4 is an innovative dental implant technique that allows for the placement of a full arch of teeth (upper or lower) using only four strategically positioned implants. It offers a fixed, stable solution for individuals with significant tooth loss or edentulism.

While treatment options exist for hair loss and tooth loss, prevention remains the best approach to maintaining optimal health and preserving natural appearance.

For hair loss prevention:

- Maintain a balanced diet: Consume a diet rich in essential nutrients such as vitamins, minerals, protein, and healthy fats to support hair growth and follicle health.

- Practice stress management: Chronic stress can contribute to hair loss by disrupting hormonal balance and increasing inflammation. Incorporate relaxation techniques such as meditation, yoga, and deep breathing exercises into your daily routine.

- Avoid harsh styling practices: Excessive heat styling, chemical treatments, and tight hairstyles can damage hair follicles and contribute to hair breakage and loss. Opt for gentler styling methods and avoid over-manipulation.

For tooth loss prevention:

- Maintain good oral hygiene by brushing your teeth twice a day, flossing daily, and incorporating oil pulling into your routine.

- Visit your dentist regularly for check-ups and cleanings to monitor your oral health.

- Avoid smoking and tobacco products, as they can increase the risk of gum disease and tooth loss.

CHAPTER 21: GENETIC TESTING & DETOXING FOR CHILDREN

In recent years, more medical regulatory groups and healthcare organizations have advocated for expanded genetic testing, particularly for newborns. Genetic testing at birth can help identify genetic conditions early, allowing for prompt intervention and treatment to improve outcomes for affected infants.

Genetic testing enables personalized healthcare approaches by providing information about a child's genetic predispositions, allowing for tailored prevention and treatment strategies.

Screening newborns for genetic conditions can have public health benefits by reducing morbidity and mortality associated with preventable genetic disorders and facilitating early intervention programs.

Advances in genetic testing technologies, such as next-generation sequencing, have made testing more accessible, affordable, and comprehensive, making it feasible to screen for a broader range of genetic conditions in newborns.

With the increasing availability and accuracy of genetic

testing, there is growing push to offer newborn screening for a wider range of genetic conditions to ensure equitable access to early diagnosis and intervention.

Many medical regulatory groups, including the American Academy of Pediatrics (AAP) and the American College of Medical Genetics and Genomics (ACMG), have issued guidelines and recommendations supporting expanded newborn screening using genetic testing technologies.

These efforts aim to improve the health outcomes of newborns and promote the integration of genetic information into routine clinical care.

△△△

Detoxification, once a practice associated primarily with adults seeking to cleanse their bodies of toxins, has gained traction in recent years as a means of supporting children's health and well-being. With increasing exposure to environmental pollutants, processed foods, and digital screens, children face unique challenges that can impact their developing bodies and minds.

Let's go through the importance of detoxing children, common toxins they may encounter, and practical strategies for supporting their natural detoxification processes.

Children are more vulnerable to the effects of toxins due to their rapid growth and development, immature detoxification systems, and increased exposure to environmental pollutants.

Toxins can disrupt various physiological processes, leading to a range of health issues, including allergies, asthma, ADHD, autism spectrum disorders, and developmental delays.

By supporting their bodies' natural detoxification pathways, we can help reduce the burden of toxins and promote optimal health and development in children.

Common toxins in children include:

- Environmental Pollutants: Children may be exposed to air pollutants, such as vehicle emissions and industrial pollutants, as well as indoor pollutants, including volatile organic compounds (VOCs) from household products and mold.
- Pesticides and Herbicides: Residues from pesticides and herbicides used in agriculture can be found on fruits, vegetables, and grains, increasing children's exposure to harmful chemicals.
- Heavy Metals: Lead, mercury, arsenic, and cadmium are examples of heavy metals that can accumulate in the body over time, potentially causing neurological and developmental disorders.
- Food Additives and Preservatives: Artificial colors, flavors, preservatives, and other additives commonly found in processed foods may adversely affect children's health, including hyperactivity and allergic reactions.
- Electronic Devices: Excessive screen time and exposure to electromagnetic radiation from electronic devices have been linked to sleep disturbances, behavioral issues, and cognitive impairments in children.

Strategies for detoxing children include:

- Clean Eating: Emphasize a diet rich in whole, organic foods, including fruits, vegetables, lean proteins, and whole grains. Minimize processed foods, sugary snacks, and artificial additives.

- Hydration: Encourage children to drink plenty of water throughout the day to support kidney function and flush out toxins from the body.

- Organic Produce: Choose organic fruits and vegetables whenever possible to reduce exposure to pesticides and herbicides.

- Safe Household Products: Opt for non-toxic cleaning supplies, personal care products, and home furnishings to minimize indoor air pollution.

- Outdoor Play: Promote outdoor play and physical activity to support respiratory health and reduce exposure to indoor pollutants.

- Mindful Screen Time: Limit screen time and encourage activities that promote creativity, physical movement, and social interaction.

- Adequate Sleep: Ensure children get enough restorative sleep each night to support detoxification and overall well-being.

- Supportive Supplements: Consider supplements such as probiotics, omega-3 fatty acids, vitamin D, and antioxidants to support immune function and detoxification pathways.

- Detox Baths: Add Epsom salts, baking soda, or essential oils to bathwater to promote relaxation and detoxification through the skin.

- Emotional Support: Create a nurturing environment with plenty of love, support, and positive reinforcement to help children cope with stress and emotional challenges.

Detoxing children is an essential aspect of promoting their health and well-being in today's increasingly toxic world. By implementing practical strategies to reduce their exposure to toxins and support their natural detoxification processes, we can help children thrive and reach their full potential. Remember, small changes can make a big difference in safeguarding the health of our children now and in the future.

My nephews are both special needs, and my sister and I have carefully detoxed them together with great success. My older nephew Tristan has cystic fibrosis (CF). CF is a genetic disorder characterized by the buildup of thick, sticky mucus in the lungs and digestive system, leading to respiratory and digestive complications.

My younger nephew Winston is autistic. Autism is a developmental disorder that affects communication, social interaction, and behavior, often characterized by repetitive behaviors and difficulty in understanding social cues.

When my sister stopped breastfeeding, she moved my nephews to a goat's milk formula at my strong recommendation. Goat's milk formula benefits kids due to its similar molecular structure to human breast milk, potentially making it easier to digest and absorb essential nutrients.

Goat's milk is rich in protein, calcium, vitamin D, riboflavin (vitamin B2), phosphorus, potassium, magnesium, vitamin B12, folate, vitamin A, zinc, and selenium, making it a nutritious option for children.

Early on, Tristan had bowel movement issues and was frequently constipated. When he was two years old, he became extremely backed up. He didn't have a bowel movement for days, became lethargic, and a fever started.

My sister took him to the hospital where she met with the surgeon who operated on him at birth to clear his intestine and reconnect it to his rectum. The intestine is connected to the rectum through the large intestine, specifically, the final portion known as the sigmoid colon, which leads to the rectum, where stool is stored before being expelled through the anus during a bowel movement.

Cystic fibrosis (CF) babies sometimes undergo a procedure known as a meconium ileus (MI) to address intestinal blockages caused by thick, sticky meconium (the baby's first stool) due to CF-related mucus buildup. This procedure involves the surgical removal of the obstructed portion of the intestine to allow for proper digestion and stool passage.

The surgeon said it was scarring tissue, and he needed an operation. My sister called me. I told her to ask for a second opinion.

"Do an enema," I said.

"We tried. It's not working," she told me.

I got all my essential oils and carrier oils and booked it to the hospital. I applied a generous amount of the mixture to his stomach and feet. Within 15-20 minutes, Tristan had a bowel movement.

Minutes later, the second opinion doctor came in with the surgeon.

"Well, doctor, I'm afraid I will have to disagree with the surgery since the patient has had a bowel movement. It's not scar tissue," he said.

Since then, my sister put him on a liquid anti-parasitic and manuka honey.

My other nephew, Winston, was nonverbal until age 4. He wasn't meeting the language and speech milestones Tristan was at that age. I told my sister I thought he was autistic.

Of course, that's hard to hear as a mother, but she agreed to start him on a zeolite spray. He was on this spray for one year, and a few months before his 5th birthday, he was having conversations with us.

Autism spectrum disorder (ASD), heavy metal toxicity, and mutations in the methylation gene group can intersect as potential factors influencing neurodevelopmental processes. Some research suggests that impaired methylation pathways and toxic heavy metal exposure may contribute to the development or severity of ASD symptoms.

I did a DNA swab analysis for my nephews. They both have mutations or deletions on the same genes that I have in my methylation, inflammation response, detoxification, and oxidative stress groups.

This genetic information has been incredibly helpful in choosing which homeopathic and naturopathic methods and remedies to utilize for their care. In addition to helping my own nephews, I've helped my cousins' children and clients' children detox with amazing results.

It's important to consult with a practitioner before giving any detox supplements to children, as their safety and appropriate dosages can vary based on factors such as age, weight, and overall health.

Some supplements that are generally considered safe for

children when taken as directed include:

- Multivitamins: Designed to provide a combination of essential vitamins and minerals, multivitamins can help fill in any nutritional gaps in a child's diet.

- Vitamin D: Especially important for bone health and immune function, vitamin D supplementation may be recommended for children who are deficient or at risk of deficiency, particularly those with limited sun exposure.

- Omega-3 fatty acids: Omega-3 supplements, such as fish oil or algae oil, can support brain development, cognitive function, and overall health in children.

- Probiotics: These beneficial bacteria can help support digestive health and strengthen the immune system, potentially reducing the risk of gastrointestinal issues and infections.

- Iron: Iron supplements may be recommended for children with iron deficiency anemia or those at risk of deficiency, such as exclusively breastfed infants or children with certain medical conditions.

- Calcium: Important for bone and teeth development, calcium supplements may be recommended for children who do not consume enough calcium-rich foods in their diet.

- Vitamin C: Known for its immune-boosting properties, vitamin C supplements may help support the immune system and reduce the duration and severity of colds and other infections in children.

It's important to choose supplements specifically formulated for children and to follow dosing instructions carefully. Additionally, parents should be aware of potential interactions between supplements and any medications their child may be taking.

CHAPTER 22: MTHFR & PREGNANT MOMS

The MTHFR gene provides instructions for producing an enzyme called methylenetetrahydrofolate reductase. This enzyme plays a crucial role in the body's methylation process, which is involved in various essential functions such as DNA synthesis, repair, and regulation, as well as the metabolism of homocysteine, an amino acid.

There are two common variants or alleles of the MTHFR gene that have been extensively studied:

C677T ALLELE

This variant involves a change at position 677 in the MTHFR gene, where a cytosine (C) is replaced by a thymine (T). Individuals who carry one or two copies of the T allele have reduced enzyme activity, leading to decreased conversion of the amino acid homocysteine to methionine. Decreased methionine can result in elevated levels of homocysteine in the blood.

A1298C ALLELE

This variant involves a change at position 1298 in the MTHFR gene, where an adenine (A) is replaced by a cytosine (C). Similar to the C677T allele, individuals who carry one or two copies of the C allele may also have reduced enzyme activity. However, the effect may be less pronounced than the C677T variant. This allele is also associated with alterations in folate metabolism and methylation processes.

Carrying one or more copies of these MTHFR gene variants may impact an individual's risk for various health conditions, including cardiovascular disease, neural tube defects, pregnancy complications, mental health disorders, and certain cancers. It's essential to note that the relationship between MTHFR gene variants and health outcomes is still complex.

The prevalence of MTHFR gene mutations or deletions varies among different populations and ethnic groups. However, it's estimated that a significant portion of the global population carries at least one copy of a common MTHFR gene variant.

For example, the C677T variant is relatively common, with studies suggesting that approximately 30% to 40% of individuals of European descent carry one copy of the T allele, and around 10% to 15% carry two copies. Similarly, the A1298C variant is also prevalent, although it may occur at lower frequencies than the C677T variant.

It's important to note that the prevalence of MTHFR gene mutations or deletions can vary widely among different populations and geographic regions. Within the U.S., Hispanics are the most impacted, according to the CDC. Less common variants or mutations within the MTHFR gene group may also exist, further contributing to genetic diversity and variability in populations.

△△△

Pregnant women with MTHFR gene mutations may have an increased risk of miscarriage due to several factors:

- Methylation Issues: MTHFR mutations can impair the body's ability to methylate properly, which is crucial for various biological processes, including DNA synthesis and hormone regulation. Methylation plays a vital role in fetal development, and disruptions in this process can increase the risk of pregnancy complications, including miscarriage.

- Homocysteine Levels: MTHFR mutations can lead to elevated levels of homocysteine, an amino acid associated with inflammation and blood vessel damage. High homocysteine levels have been linked to an increased risk of miscarriage and pregnancy complications.

- Folate Metabolism: MTHFR mutations can affect the metabolism of folate, a B vitamin essential for fetal development. Inadequate folate levels due to impaired metabolism can lead to neural tube defects and other pregnancy complications that may result in miscarriage.

To help prevent miscarriage in pregnant women with MTHFR mutations, several strategies can be implemented:

- Supplementation: It's essential for pregnant

women with MTHFR mutations to supplement with methyl folate, the active form of folate that bypasses the impaired enzyme function associated with MTHFR mutations. Methyl folate supplementation can help support healthy fetal development and reduce the risk of miscarriage.

- B vitamins: In addition to methyl folate, pregnant women with MTHFR mutations may benefit from supplementation with other B vitamins, such as B6 and B12, which play a role in methylation and homocysteine metabolism.

- Antioxidants: Antioxidants like vitamin C, vitamin E, and selenium can help reduce oxidative stress and inflammation associated with elevated homocysteine levels and MTHFR mutations, potentially lowering the risk of miscarriage.

- Healthy Lifestyle: Maintaining a healthy lifestyle, including a balanced diet, regular exercise, adequate sleep, and stress management, is crucial for supporting overall health and reducing the risk of pregnancy complications.

- Regular Prenatal Care: Pregnant women with MTHFR mutations should receive regular prenatal care and work closely with healthcare providers to monitor pregnancy progression and address any potential complications promptly.

To develop a personalized care plan tailored to specific needs and circumstances, other genes in the methylation group must be assessed.

These include:

- COMT (Catechol-O-Methyltransferase): COMT is

involved in the breakdown of catecholamines, such as dopamine, epinephrine, and norepinephrine. Variants in the COMT gene can affect the enzyme's activity, leading to differences in neurotransmitter levels and impacting mood, cognition, and stress response.

- MTR (5-Methyltetrahydrofolate-Homocysteine Methyltransferase): MTR plays a key role in the conversion of homocysteine to methionine, a process that requires methyl cobalamin (vitamin B12) as a cofactor. Variants in the MTR gene can affect this conversion, leading to elevated homocysteine levels and potentially increasing the risk of cardiovascular disease and other health problems.

- MTRR (5-Methyltetrahydrofolate-Homocysteine Methyltransferase Reductase): MTRR is involved in the regeneration of methyl cobalamin, the active form of vitamin B12, which is necessary for the conversion of homocysteine to methionine. Variants in the MTRR gene can impair this process, leading to reduced levels of methyl cobalamin and elevated homocysteine levels.

- BHMT (Betaine-Homocysteine Methyltransferase): BHMT is involved in an alternative pathway for homocysteine metabolism, using betaine as a methyl donor to convert homocysteine to methionine. Variants in the BHMT gene can affect this pathway, impacting methionine synthesis and potentially contributing to elevated homocysteine levels.

- CBS (Cystathionine Beta-Synthase): CBS is involved in the conversion of homocysteine to cystathionine, a process that requires vitamin B6 (pyridoxal phosphate) as a cofactor. Variants in the CBS gene can impair this conversion, leading to elevated homocysteine levels and potentially increasing the risk of cardiovascular disease and other health problems.

These genes collectively play critical roles in the methylation pathway, which is involved in numerous biological processes, including DNA synthesis and repair, neurotransmitter metabolism, hormone regulation, and detoxification.

Variants in these genes can impact methylation processes, potentially leading to health issues and increasing susceptibility to various conditions. Understanding individual genetic variations can provide valuable insights for personalized health management and treatment strategies.

MTHFR genetic mutations or deletions have been implicated in playing an underlying role in a variety of diseases and conditions.

Some of these include:

- Cardiovascular disease: MTHFR mutations are associated with elevated homocysteine levels, which can contribute to an increased risk of cardiovascular disease, including coronary artery disease, stroke, and venous thromboembolism.

- Neural tube defects: MTHFR mutations are linked to impaired folate metabolism, which can increase the risk of neural tube defects such as spina bifida and anencephaly in newborns.

- Pregnancy complications: MTHFR mutations have been associated with an increased risk of pregnancy complications, including recurrent miscarriages, preeclampsia, and preterm birth.

- Mental health disorders: MTHFR mutations may be associated with an increased risk of mental health disorders such as depression, anxiety, bipolar disorder, and schizophrenia.

- Cancer: MTHFR mutations have been implicated in various types of cancer, including colorectal cancer, breast cancer, prostate cancer, and leukemia, although the relationship is complex and not fully understood.

- Neurological disorders: MTHFR mutations have been linked to neurodevelopmental disorders such as autism spectrum disorder and attention deficit hyperactivity disorder (ADHD), as well as neurodegenerative diseases such as Alzheimer's disease and Parkinson's disease.

- Chronic conditions: MTHFR mutations may contribute to the development or progression of chronic conditions such as fibromyalgia, chronic fatigue syndrome, irritable bowel syndrome (IBS), and migraines.

While MTHFR mutations may play a role in certain diseases and conditions, they are also influenced by a number of factors.

The impact of MTHFR mutations on disease risk can vary depending on the specific mutation, other genetic variations, lifestyle factors, and overall health status.

Therefore, interpretation of genetic testing results and management of associated health risks should be done in consultation with a qualified healthcare professional.

CHAPTER 23: CELLULAR FUNCTIONALITY & THE CELL CYCLE

The processes that occur within individual cells are referred to as cellular-level functionality. We are only made up of cells and energy.

These include metabolism, energy production, protein synthesis, signaling pathways, and maintenance of cellular structures and functions. Cellular processes are essential for overall health and are tightly regulated to ensure proper functioning of tissues, organs, and systems within the body.

Cellular processes help maintain internal balance and stability (homeostasis) by regulating various physiological parameters such as pH, temperature, and nutrient levels. These processes play a crucial role in tissue repair, wound healing, and regeneration, ensuring the body's ability to recover from injury and maintain tissue integrity.

Cells generate energy through processes like cellular respiration and ATP production, which is necessary for supporting essential functions and activities throughout the body.

Cellular signaling pathways allow cells to communicate with each other and coordinate responses to internal and external stimuli, enabling proper physiological responses and adaptation.

When cellular processes are disrupted or dysfunctional, it can lead to various health problems and diseases, including metabolic disorders, immune system dysfunction, neurodegenerative diseases, cancer, and cardiovascular diseases.

Dysfunction at the cellular level may result from genetic mutations, environmental factors, lifestyle choices, nutrient deficiencies, oxidative stress, inflammation, and other factors. Several genes are involved in regulating cellular processes and functions.

Here are key gene families and their functions:

> ATP Synthase Genes: Code for proteins involved in ATP synthesis, the primary energy currency of cells.

- Insulin Receptor Genes: Code for receptors that play a crucial role in glucose uptake and metabolism.
- Tumor Suppressor Genes (e.g., TP53): Code for proteins that help regulate cell growth, division, and apoptosis, preventing the development of cancer.
- Antioxidant Enzyme Genes (e.g., SOD1, CAT): Code for enzymes that protect cells from oxidative damage by scavenging free radicals.
- Cell Cycle Regulatory Genes (e.g., CDKs, cyclins): Code for proteins that control the progression of

the cell cycle, ensuring accurate cell replication and division.

A balanced diet rich in vitamins, minerals, antioxidants, essential fatty acids, and amino acids is essential for maintaining cellular health and function.

Examples of nutrients important for cellular function include:

- Antioxidants: Vitamin C, vitamin E, selenium, and flavonoids help protect cells from oxidative stress and damage.
- Essential Fatty Acids: Omega-3 and omega-6 fatty acids are important for maintaining cell membrane integrity and function.
- Micronutrients: Minerals such as magnesium, zinc, and iron are essential cofactors for various cellular enzymes and processes.
- Protein: Amino acids from dietary protein sources are necessary for protein synthesis, cell repair, and tissue regeneration.

Nutrients obtained from whole foods are often more bioavailable and better utilized by the body than those obtained from synthetic supplements. Whole foods contain a complex matrix of nutrients, phytochemicals, and fiber that synergistically support cellular health and overall well-being.

Synthetic supplements may provide isolated nutrients in concentrated forms, but they may lack the full spectrum of compounds found in whole foods and may not have the same health benefits.

Excessive intake of certain synthetic supplements may have adverse effects or interact with medications. In contrast, nutrients from whole foods are generally considered safe when consumed as part of a balanced diet.

Maintaining optimal cellular function is crucial for overall health and well-being. Proper nutrition, lifestyle choices, and environmental factors play key roles in supporting cellular health, while dysfunction at the cellular level can contribute to various health problems and diseases.

Choosing nutrient-rich foods and adopting healthy lifestyle habits are essential for promoting optimal cellular function and preventing cellular dysfunction.

The life cycle of a cell, known as the cell cycle, is a series of stages that a cell goes through as it grows, prepares for division, divides, and then eventually undergoes cell death (apoptosis).

Cell death plays an important roles in maintaining tissue homeostasis and eliminating damaged or dysfunctional cells. However, dysregulation of cell death pathways can contribute to various diseases, including cancer, neurodegenerative disorders, autoimmune diseases, and ischemic injuries.

Understanding the mechanisms and regulation of cell death is essential for developing therapies to target specific cell death pathways and treat diseases associated with abnormal cell death or survival.

Cell death is important for several reasons:

- Tissue Homeostasis: Cell death, particularly programmed cell death (apoptosis), is crucial for maintaining tissue homeostasis by eliminating damaged, aged, or unwanted cells. This process ensures the efficient removal of cells that are no longer functional or necessary for the proper functioning of tissues and organs.

- Development and Growth: During development, cell death plays a vital role in sculpting tissues and organs by removing excess cells and refining their structures. This process, known as developmental apoptosis, helps shape the formation of organs and tissues and ensures their proper function.

- Immune Response: Cell death is involved in the body's immune response to infections and disease. Infected or damaged cells can undergo programmed cell death to limit the spread of pathogens and trigger immune responses for their clearance.

- Prevention of Disease: Dysregulated cell death processes can contribute to the development of various diseases, including cancer, autoimmune disorders, and neurodegenerative diseases. Understanding the mechanisms of cell death and its regulation is essential for developing therapies to target specific pathways and treat these conditions.

New cells are continuously created in the body through a process called cell proliferation. Cell proliferation involves the division of existing cells to produce daughter cells, which then mature and differentiate into various cell types to replace old, damaged, or dying cells. This process occurs in tissues with high turnover rates, such as the skin, gastrointestinal tract, bone marrow, and blood cells.

In tissues with lower turnover rates, such as the heart and brain, cell proliferation may be limited, and the replacement of cells may occur at a slower pace or may be less frequent. However, stem cells and progenitor cells in these tissues can still contribute to cell renewal and repair under certain conditions or in response to injury or disease.

CHAPTER 24: NUTRIENT DEFICIENT FOOD & SUPPLEMENTS

Nutrient and mineral-deficient foods have become increasingly prevalent in modern diets, posing significant health concerns for populations worldwide. Several factors contribute to this decline in nutrient density, including changes in agricultural practices, food processing methods, and dietary trends.

These include:

- Agricultural Practices: Intensive farming practices, including monocropping and the use of synthetic fertilizers, have depleted soil quality and reduced the nutrient content of crops. Over time, this degradation of soil health has led to diminished levels of essential vitamins, minerals, and phytonutrients in fruits, vegetables, grains, and other agricultural products.

- Food Processing: The widespread adoption of industrial food processing techniques has further exacerbated nutrient loss in foods. Processes such as milling, refining, and cooking can strip away valuable nutrients, including fiber, vitamins, and minerals, from whole foods, leaving behind refined products with lower nutritional value.

- Dietary Trends: Shifts in dietary patterns towards processed, convenience foods high in sugar, salt, and unhealthy fats have contributed to nutrient deficiencies in populations. These highly processed foods often lack essential nutrients while being loaded with empty calories and additives, leading to imbalances in nutrient intake and increased risk of chronic diseases.

Many modern diets are characterized by an overabundance of processed and nutrient-deficient foods. These foods often contain excessive amounts of refined carbohydrates, added sugars, unhealthy fats, and sodium, which can displace nutrient-rich whole foods and contribute to nutritional imbalances and other deficiencies.

To address these concerns and support optimal health and well-being, it is essential to prioritize nutrient-dense foods that provide a wide array of essential vitamins, minerals, antioxidants, and phytonutrients.

Some key nutrients and minerals that are crucial for proper bodily function and should be obtained from food and water daily include:

- Protein: Essential for muscle growth and repair, hormone synthesis, and immune function.
- Omega-3 fatty acids: Important for brain health, heart health, and inflammation regulation.
- Fiber: Supports digestive health, regulates blood sugar levels, and promotes satiety.
- Vitamin A: Essential for vision, immune function,

and skin health.

- Vitamin C: Acts as an antioxidant, supports immune function, and aids in collagen synthesis.
- Vitamin D: Crucial for bone health, immune function, and mood regulation.
- Calcium: Necessary for bone and teeth health, muscle function, and nerve transmission.
- Iron: Required for oxygen transport, energy production, and immune function.
- Magnesium: Involved in hundreds of biochemical reactions in the body, including energy metabolism, muscle function, and bone health.
- Potassium: Important for fluid balance, muscle contractions, and nerve transmission.

Ensuring adequate hydration and access to clean, mineral-rich water sources is just as essential, because water plays a crucial role in virtually every bodily function.

Seeking out specific types of supplements, such as whole food cold-pressed plant-based supplements and liposomal supplements, is important for several reasons.

These include:

- Nutrient Bioavailability: Whole food cold-pressed plant-based supplements are derived from natural foods, which means they contain the full spectrum of nutrients found in nature. These supplements retain the natural synergy and bioavailability of nutrients, making it easier for the body to recognize and absorb them than synthetic alternatives. Liposomal supplements utilize lipid-based delivery systems to encapsulate nutrients, enhancing their absorption and bioavailability by protecting them from degradation in the digestive tract.

- Nutrient Quality: Whole food supplements are made from minimally processed, nutrient-rich plant foods, preserving their natural nutritional content. Cold-pressed extraction methods involve minimal heat and mechanical processing, which helps retain the integrity of delicate nutrients like vitamins, minerals, enzymes, and phytonutrients. In contrast, synthetic supplements are often isolated nutrients produced through chemical synthesis, lacking the complex matrix of co-factors and phytochemicals present in whole foods.

- Avoidance of Synthetic Fillers: Whole food supplements and liposomal supplements typically avoid synthetic fillers, binders, and excipients commonly found in conventional supplements. These additives are used to improve shelf life, aid in manufacturing, or enhance appearance. Still, they may have little to no nutritional value and could potentially cause adverse reactions in sensitive individuals.

- Health Benefits: Whole food supplements and liposomal supplements are often associated with a range of health benefits, including enhanced nutrient absorption, improved cellular function, and better overall health outcomes. By providing nutrients in their natural form and optimal delivery systems, these supplements may support various aspects of health, including immune function, antioxidant defense, energy metabolism, and tissue repair.

Choosing whole food cold-pressed plant-based supplements and liposomal supplements over other options ensures that you obtain high-quality, bioavailable nutrients that closely resemble those found in nature.

While these supplements may come at a slightly higher cost, their potential health benefits and superior nutrient profiles make them a worthwhile investment in your overall well-being.

△△△

Understanding the roles of amino acids, hormones, neurotransmitters, vitamins, minerals, and positive metals (cations) is essential for maintaining optimal health and function.

Amino acids are the building blocks of proteins. Hormones regulate metabolism and stress response. Neurotransmitters influence mood and cognitive function. Vitamins and minerals support various physiological processes. And, positive metals play critical roles in fluid balance, nerve transmission, and muscle function.

Here's your top 10 for each:

AMINO ACIDS

- Glutamine: Supports immune function, aids in gut health, promotes muscle repair, and serves as a precursor for other amino acids and molecules.
- Leucine: Stimulates protein synthesis, supports muscle growth and repair, and regulates blood

sugar levels.

- Lysine: Essential for collagen formation, tissue repair, and the production of enzymes, hormones, and antibodies.

- Valine: Important for muscle metabolism, tissue repair, and the maintenance of nitrogen balance in the body.

- Isoleucine: Supports muscle metabolism, energy production, and the regulation of blood sugar levels.

- Methionine: A precursor for other amino acids and important for protein synthesis, as well as to produce antioxidants and various molecules involved in detoxification.

- Phenylalanine: Precursor for the synthesis of neurotransmitters like dopamine, norepinephrine, and epinephrine, and important for mood regulation and cognitive function.

- Threonine: Essential for protein synthesis and important for the formation of collagen, elastin, and other structural proteins.

- Tryptophan: Precursor for the synthesis of serotonin, a neurotransmitter involved in mood regulation, sleep, and appetite.

- Histidine: Precursor for the synthesis of histamine, an important neurotransmitter involved in immune response and allergic reactions.

ENZYMES

- ATP synthase: Catalyzes the synthesis of ATP from ADP and inorganic phosphate during cellular respiration.
- Catalase: Catalyzes the decomposition of hydrogen peroxide into water and oxygen, protecting cells from oxidative damage.
- DNA polymerase: Catalyzes the synthesis of new DNA strands during DNA replication and repair.
- Ribonuclease: Catalyzes the degradation of RNA molecules into smaller components.
- Protease: Catalyzes the breakdown of proteins into amino acids.
- Lipase: Catalyzes the breakdown of lipids into fatty acids and glycerol.
- Amylase: Catalyzes the breakdown of starch and glycogen into smaller carbohydrate molecules.
- Kinase: Catalyzes the transfer of phosphate groups from ATP to other molecules, regulating various cellular processes.
- Phosphatase: Catalyzes the removal of phosphate groups from proteins, regulating their activity.
- Helicase: Catalyzes the unwinding of DNA double helix during DNA replication and repair.

HORMONES

- Insulin: Regulates blood sugar levels by glucose uptake into cells and storing excess glucose as glycogen.

- Cortisol: Regulates metabolism, immune response, and stress response.
- Thyroid hormone (T3 and T4): Regulates metabolism, growth, and development.
- Testosterone: Regulates male reproductive functions, muscle mass, and bone density.
- Estrogen: Regulates female reproductive functions, bone density, and cardiovascular health.
- Growth hormone: Stimulates growth, cell reproduction, and regeneration.
- Adrenaline (epinephrine): Triggers the body's fight-or-flight response, increasing heart rate, blood pressure, and energy availability.
- Melatonin: Regulates sleep-wake cycles and has antioxidant properties.
- Glucagon: Raises blood sugar levels by promoting the breakdown of glycogen and the release of glucose from the liver.
- Parathyroid hormone (PTH): Regulates calcium and phosphate levels in the blood and bone remodeling.

NEUROTRANSMITTERS

- Serotonin: Regulates mood, appetite, sleep, and cognitive function.
- Dopamine: Involved in reward-motivated behavior, motor control, and mood regulation.

- Acetylcholine: Involved in muscle contraction, memory, and attention.

- Gamma-aminobutyric acid (GABA): Acts as an inhibitory neurotransmitter, reducing neuronal excitability and promoting relaxation.

- Glutamate: Acts as an excitatory neurotransmitter, involved in learning, memory, and synaptic plasticity.

- Norepinephrine: Involved in the body's fight-or-flight response, regulating arousal, attention, and mood.

- Endorphins: Act as natural pain relievers and are associated with feelings of pleasure and euphoria.

- Histamine: Involved in immune response, allergic reactions, and neurotransmission in the brain.

- Glycine: Acts as an inhibitory neurotransmitter in the spinal cord and brainstem, regulating muscle tone and reflexes.

- Adenosine: Regulates sleep-wake cycles and promotes relaxation by inhibiting neurotransmitter release.

NUTRIENTS

- Water: Essential for hydration, nutrient transport, and various physiological processes.

- Carbohydrates: Main source of energy for the body, particularly glucose.

- Proteins: Important for tissue repair, muscle

growth, enzyme production, and immune function.

- Fats: Provide energy and insulation and serve as structural components of cell membranes.

- Vitamins (C, D, B12, A, E, K, B6, B9, B1, B2): Essential for metabolism, immune function, and overall health.

- Fiber: Aids digestion, regulates bowel movements, and promotes gut health.

- Minerals (calcium, magnesium, potassium, sodium, phosphorus, chloride, iron, zinc, copper, manganese): Essential for various physiological functions, including bone health, muscle function, and electrolyte balance.

- Antioxidants: Help protect cells from damage caused by free radicals, reducing the risk of chronic diseases.

- Omega-3 fatty acids: Support heart health, brain function, and inflammation regulation.

- Phytonutrients: Found in plant-based foods, these compounds have antioxidant and anti-inflammatory properties, supporting overall health.

POSITIVE METALS

- Sodium (Na^+): Regulates fluid balance, nerve function, and muscle contraction.

- Potassium (K^+): Important for fluid balance, nerve transmission, and muscle contraction.

- Calcium (Ca^{2+}): Essential for bone and teeth health, muscle function, and nerve transmission.

- Magnesium (Mg^{2+}): Involved in over 300 enzymatic processes, supports muscle and nerve function and energy metabolism.

- Iron (Fe^{2+}): Critical for oxygen transport, energy production, and enzyme function.

- Zinc (Zn^{2+}): Important for immune function, wound healing, and protein synthesis.

- Copper (Cu^{2+}): Necessary for iron metabolism, connective tissue formation, and antioxidant function.

- Manganese (Mn^{2+}): Supports bone health, metabolism, and antioxidant defenses.

- Cobalt (Co^{2+}): Essential component of vitamin B12, involved in DNA synthesis and red blood cell formation.

- Nickel (Ni^{2+}): Plays a role in certain enzymatic reactions and may have a role in the body's immune response.

MINERALS

- Calcium: Essential for bone and teeth health, muscle function, and nerve transmission.

- Magnesium: Involved in over 300 enzymatic processes, supports muscle and nerve function, and energy metabolism.

- Potassium: Important for fluid balance, nerve

transmission, and muscle contraction.

- Sodium: Regulates fluid balance, nerve function, and muscle contraction.
- Phosphorus: Essential for bone and teeth health, energy metabolism, and cell structure.
- Chloride: Helps maintain fluid balance, stomach acid production, and nerve function.
- Iron: Critical for oxygen transport, energy production, and enzyme function.
- Zinc: Important for immune function, wound healing, and protein synthesis.
- Copper: Necessary for iron metabolism, connective tissue formation, and antioxidant function.
- Manganese: Supports bone health, metabolism, and antioxidant defenses.

VITAMINS

- Vitamin C (ascorbic acid): Important for immune function, collagen synthesis, and antioxidant activity.
- Vitamin D: Essential for bone health, calcium absorption, and immune function.
- Vitamin B12 (cobalamin): Necessary for red blood cell formation, nerve function, and DNA synthesis.
- Vitamin A: Important for vision, immune function, and skin health.
- Vitamin E: Acts as an antioxidant, protecting cells

from damage caused by free radicals.

- Vitamin K: Essential for blood clotting and bone health.

- Vitamin B6 (pyridoxine): Involved in amino acid metabolism, neurotransmitter synthesis, and immune function.

- Folate (vitamin B9): Important for DNA synthesis, cell division, and red blood cell formation.

- Vitamin B1 (thiamine): Essential for energy metabolism and nerve function.

- Vitamin B2 (riboflavin): Involved in energy production, metabolism, and antioxidant activity.

CHAPTER 25: SUPER SUPPLEMENTS, COMBINATIONS, & RX INTERACTIONS

There has been a growing interest in natural remedies and supplements for promoting health and well-being that provide high concentrations of mineral content for a "super" effect.

Supplements that have gained popularity for their potential health benefits are sea moss, moringa, and black seed oil. Each offers a unique combination of vitamins, minerals, and other bioactive compounds that can support overall health.

SEA MOSS

Also known as Irish moss or carrageenan moss, is a type of seaweed that grows in coastal regions around the world. It has been used for centuries in traditional medicine for its purported health benefits.

Sea moss is rich in essential minerals, vitamins, and

antioxidants, making it a popular choice for supporting overall health and well-being.

It can be consumed in various forms, including dried, powdered, or as a gel. It can be added to smoothies, soups, and sauces or used as a thickening agent in recipes. The recommended dosage varies depending on individual health needs.

Benefits include:

- Rich in Iodine: Sea moss is an excellent source of iodine, a mineral that is essential for thyroid function and metabolism regulation.

- Contains Calcium and Magnesium: These minerals are important for bone health, muscle function, and nerve transmission.

- High in Iron: Iron is necessary for the production of red blood cells and oxygen transport in the body.

- Provides Potassium: Potassium is crucial for heart health, muscle function, and electrolyte balance.

- Contains Zinc: Zinc supports immune function, wound healing, and cell growth.

MORINGA

Also known as the "miracle tree," is a nutrient-dense plant native to parts of Africa and Asia. It has been used for centuries in traditional medicine for its potential health-promoting properties.

Moringa is rich in vitamins, minerals, antioxidants, and bioactive compounds, making it a popular choice for supporting overall health and vitality.

Moringa can be consumed as a powder, capsules, or brewed as a tea. It can be added to smoothies, salads, and soups or used as a seasoning for various dishes. The recommended dosage may vary, but starting with 1-2 teaspoons of moringa powder per day is common.

Benefits include:

- High in Calcium: Moringa contains calcium, which is essential for bone health and muscle function.
- Rich in Iron: Iron is important for oxygen transport in the body and preventing iron-deficiency anemia.
- Contains Magnesium: Magnesium supports nerve function, muscle relaxation, and energy production.
- Provides Potassium: Potassium is crucial for heart health, blood pressure regulation, and electrolyte balance.
- Rich in Zinc: Zinc supports immune function, wound healing, and DNA synthesis.

BLACK SEED OIL

Also referred to as Nigella sativa oil or black cumin seed oil, this has been used for centuries in traditional medicine for its potential health benefits.

It is derived from the seeds of the Nigella sativa plant, which is native to South Asia. Black seed oil is rich in essential fatty acids, vitamins, minerals, and antioxidants, making it a popular choice for supporting overall health and well-being.

Black seed oil can be consumed orally or applied topically. It can be ingested directly, added to smoothies and salads, or used as a dressing for dishes. The recommended dosage may vary, but starting with 1-2 teaspoons of black seed oil per day is common.

It is important to choose high-quality, cold-pressed black seed oil for optimal benefits.

Benefits include:

- Contains Magnesium: Magnesium supports nerve function, muscle relaxation, and energy production.
- Provides Calcium: Calcium is essential for bone health, muscle function, and nerve transmission.
- Rich in Iron: Iron is necessary for red blood cell production and oxygen transport in the body.
- Contains Potassium: Potassium is crucial for heart health, blood pressure regulation, and electrolyte balance.
- Provides Zinc: Zinc supports immune function, wound healing, and cell growth.

Other "super supplements" to consider include:

BERBERINE

This compound found in several plants, including goldenseal, barberry and oregon grape, has been studied for its potential benefits in promoting increased metabolism and weight loss.

These include:

- Regulation of Blood Sugar Levels: Berberine may help regulate blood sugar levels by increasing insulin sensitivity, which can lead to improved glucose metabolism. By stabilizing blood sugar levels, berberine may help reduce cravings and promote weight loss.

- Enhanced Fat Burning: Research suggests that berberine may activate an enzyme called AMP-activated protein kinase (AMPK), which plays a role in regulating metabolism. Activation of AMPK may increase fat burning and energy expenditure, contributing to weight loss.

- Reduced Fat Accumulation: Berberine has been shown to inhibit the growth and differentiation of fat cells, potentially reducing fat accumulation in the body. This effect may help prevent weight gain and promote weight loss.

- Improved Gut Health: Berberine has antimicrobial properties and may help balance the gut microbiota. A healthy gut microbiome is associated with improved metabolism and weight management.

- Appetite Suppression: Some studies suggest that berberine may help reduce appetite and food intake, leading to fewer calories consumed and aiding in weight loss efforts.

- Lowered Inflammation: Chronic inflammation is associated with obesity and metabolic disorders. Berberine has been found to have anti-inflammatory effects, which may contribute to its beneficial effects on metabolism and weight loss.

- Cardiometabolic Benefits: Berberine has been shown to improve lipid profiles, including lowering LDL cholesterol and triglyceride levels, which are risk factors for heart disease and metabolic syndrome. By improving overall cardiovascular health, berberine may support weight loss efforts.

BLUE VERVAIN

Also called as Verbena hastata, this herb is traditionally used to address various health issues, including anxiety.

Benefits include:

- Relaxation and Calming Effects: Blue vervain contains compounds that may have mild sedative properties, which could help promote relaxation and reduce anxiety and nervousness.

- Support for Nervous System: Blue vervain has been used historically to support the nervous system and may help soothe frazzled nerves, providing a sense of calmness and tranquility.

- Muscle Relaxation: Blue vervain may have muscle-relaxing properties, which can benefit individuals experiencing tension-related anxiety or physical symptoms of anxiety such as muscle tightness or stiffness.

- Mood Enhancement: Some herbalists believe that blue vervain may have mood-enhancing effects, potentially helping to uplift mood and alleviate feelings of depression or low mood that often accompany anxiety disorders.

- Sleep Support: By promoting relaxation and reducing anxiety, blue vervain may indirectly support better sleep quality, as anxiety is a common cause of sleep disturbances.

- Antioxidant Activity: Blue vervain contains antioxidants, which help protect the body from oxidative stress and inflammation. Chronic stress and anxiety can increase oxidative damage in the body, so antioxidant-rich herbs like blue vervain may provide additional support for overall well-being.

- Gastrointestinal Support: Anxiety can sometimes manifest with gastrointestinal symptoms such as stomach upset or irritable bowel syndrome (IBS). Blue vervain may have soothing effects on the digestive system, potentially alleviating some of these symptoms.

LION'S MANE MUSHROOM

This has gained attention for its potential health benefits, including its possible role in cancer prevention and treatment.

These include:

- Anticancer Properties: Some laboratory and animal studies have indicated that compounds found in lion's mane mushrooms, such as polysaccharides and hericenones, may have anticancer properties. These compounds have shown potential in inhibiting the growth of various cancer cell lines, including colon, gastric, and leukemia cells.

- Immune System Support: Lion's mane mushrooms contain beta-glucans and other bioactive compounds that may help modulate the immune system. A healthy immune system is crucial for identifying and eliminating cancerous cells, and lion's mane may support immune function, potentially enhancing the body's ability to fight cancer.

- Reduction of Chemotherapy Side Effects: Some studies suggest that lion's mane mushroom extract may help reduce certain side effects associated with chemotherapy and radiation therapy, such as nausea, vomiting, and neuropathy. By providing supportive care during cancer treatment, lion's mane could potentially improve patients' quality of life.

- Neuroprotective Effects: Cancer treatments, particularly chemotherapy, can sometimes lead to cognitive impairment known as "chemo brain." Lion's mane mushrooms have been studied for their potential neuroprotective effects and ability to support cognitive function. These neuroprotective effects could be beneficial for cancer patients experiencing cognitive decline during treatment.

- Anti-Inflammatory Effects: Chronic inflammation is associated with cancer development and progression. Lion's mane mushrooms contain anti-inflammatory compounds that may help reduce inflammation in the body, potentially slowing the progression of cancer and improving overall health outcomes.

- Gut Health Support: Emerging research suggests a link between gut health and cancer risk. Lion's mane mushrooms may support gut health by promoting the growth of beneficial gut bacteria and reducing inflammation in the digestive tract, which could contribute to a lower risk of certain types of cancer.

PURPLE LOTUS FLOWER

This is revered for various health benefits and cultural significance in many parts of the world.

Benefits of this flower include:

- Antioxidant Properties: Purple lotus flower contains compounds with antioxidant properties, such as flavonoids and polyphenols. These antioxidants help neutralize free radicals in the body, reducing oxidative stress and inflammation, which are linked to various chronic diseases.

- Stress Reduction: In traditional medicine systems like Ayurveda and Traditional Chinese Medicine (TCM), purple lotus flower is believed to have calming and stress-relieving properties. Consuming lotus flower tea or extract may help promote relaxation and mental well-being.

- Digestive Health: Lotus flower has been used historically to support digestive health. It may help alleviate digestive discomfort, such as bloating, gas, and indigestion. Lotus flower tea or decoctions are often consumed for their digestive benefits.

- Skin Health: Lotus flower extract is sometimes

used in skincare products due to its moisturizing and antioxidant properties. It may help hydrate the skin, improve elasticity, and protect against premature aging caused by environmental factors.

- Heart Health: Some research suggests that compounds found in lotus flower, such as flavonoids and alkaloids, may have cardioprotective effects. They may help lower blood pressure, reduce cholesterol levels, and improve overall cardiovascular health.

SARSAPARILLA

This herb has been traditionally used for various purposes, including blood purification and cleansing.

Some benefits include:

- Detoxification: Sarsaparilla contains saponins, flavonoids, and other compounds that may have detoxifying properties. It is believed that these compounds help support the liver's natural detoxification processes, potentially aiding in the removal of toxins and impurities from the blood.

- Anti-inflammatory Effects: Chronic inflammation can contribute to various health issues, including cardiovascular disease. Sarsaparilla contains anti-inflammatory compounds that may help reduce inflammation in the body, including inflammation associated with blood vessels. By reducing inflammation, sarsaparilla may support overall cardiovascular health.

- Antioxidant Activity: Sarsaparilla contains antioxidants, such as flavonoids and phenolic compounds, which help neutralize free radicals and reduce oxidative stress in the body. Oxidative stress can damage cells and contribute to various health problems, including cardiovascular disease. By scavenging free radicals, sarsaparilla may help protect blood vessels and promote overall cardiovascular health.

- Potential Antimicrobial Effects: Some studies suggest that sarsaparilla may have antimicrobial properties, which could help prevent or treat infections that affect the blood or circulatory system. By inhibiting the growth of harmful microorganisms, sarsaparilla may support overall blood health.

- Blood Sugar Regulation: High blood sugar levels can have detrimental effects on cardiovascular health and contribute to conditions such as diabetes and metabolic syndrome. Some research suggests that sarsaparilla may help regulate blood sugar levels, potentially reducing the risk of complications related to high blood sugar.

- Improved Circulation: Sarsaparilla has been traditionally used to promote healthy circulation. By supporting blood vessel health and circulation, sarsaparilla may help ensure that oxygen and nutrients are efficiently delivered to tissues throughout the body.

While these potential benefits are promising, it's important to note that scientific evidence supporting these "super" supplements is limited.

Any supplements should be used under the guidance of a healthcare professional, especially for individuals with underlying health conditions or those taking medications, as they may interact with certain drugs.

△△△

Optimizing nutrient absorption is essential for ensuring that the body can effectively utilize the vitamins, minerals, and other essential compounds obtained from dietary supplements. Some supplements work synergistically, enhancing each other's absorption and overall effectiveness.

Understanding which supplements can be combined for maximum absorption can help individuals make informed choices to support their health and well-being.

Here is a list of supplements that are commonly recommended to be taken together for optimal absorption and efficacy.

- Vitamin D and Calcium: Vitamin D enhances the absorption of calcium in the gut, promoting bone health and supporting overall skeletal strength. Taking these two supplements together can maximize calcium absorption and utilization in the body.

- Vitamin C and Iron: Vitamin C helps increase the absorption of iron from plant-based sources (non-heme iron) and enhances its bioavailability. Combining vitamin C with iron supplements or iron-rich foods can support healthy red blood cell production and prevent iron deficiency anemia.

- Vitamin K2 and Vitamin D: Vitamin K2 works synergistically with vitamin D to support bone health by directing calcium to the bones and teeth while preventing its accumulation in soft tissues. Taking vitamin K2 alongside vitamin D can enhance calcium metabolism and reduce the risk of arterial calcification.

- Magnesium and Vitamin D: Magnesium plays a crucial role in vitamin D metabolism and activation, facilitating its conversion into its active form in the body. Pairing magnesium with vitamin D can enhance vitamin D absorption and utilization, supporting bone health, muscle function, and overall well-being.

- Omega-3 Fatty Acids and Vitamin E: Vitamin E acts as an antioxidant, protecting omega-3 fatty acids from oxidation and preserving their integrity and efficacy. Taking vitamin E alongside omega-3 supplements can enhance their bioavailability and ensure optimal benefits for cardiovascular health and inflammation management.

- Probiotics and Prebiotics: Probiotics are beneficial bacteria that support gut health and digestion, while prebiotics are non-digestible fibers that serve as food for probiotics, promoting their growth and activity. Combining probiotics and prebiotics can create an optimal environment for beneficial gut bacteria, enhancing their colonization and functionality.

- Zinc and Copper: Zinc and copper have a delicate balance in the body, and taking them together in appropriate ratios can support immune function, antioxidant defense, and enzyme activity. Zinc facilitates the absorption of copper, while copper helps regulate zinc metabolism, ensuring optimal utilization of both minerals.

- Vitamin B Complex: Vitamin B complex supplements contain a combination of various B vitamins, including B1 (thiamine), B2 (riboflavin), B3 (niacin), B5 (pantothenic acid), B6 (pyridoxine), B7 (biotin), B9 (folate), and B12 (cobalamin). These vitamins work synergistically to support energy metabolism, nervous system function, and cellular health. Taking a complete B complex can ensure balanced levels of all B vitamins for optimal absorption and utilization.

- Curcumin and Piperine: Curcumin, the active compound in turmeric, has potent anti-inflammatory and antioxidant properties, but its absorption is limited. Piperine, found in black pepper, can enhance the bioavailability of curcumin by inhibiting its metabolism in the liver and intestines. Taking curcumin supplements with piperine can significantly improve curcumin absorption and efficacy.

- Vitamin A and Healthy Fats: Vitamin A is a fat-soluble vitamin that requires the presence of dietary fats for optimal absorption and utilization. Consuming vitamin A-rich foods or supplements with healthy fats, such as avocado, olive oil, or nuts, can enhance vitamin A absorption and support vision health, immune function, and skin integrity.

By understanding which supplements can be taken together for maximum absorption, individuals can optimize their nutrient intake and support their overall health and well-being.

Confer with a healthcare professional before starting any

new supplement regimen, especially if you have underlying health conditions or are taking medications. They can help to ensure safe and effective supplementation.

Dietary supplements have become increasingly popular for supporting overall well-being and addressing specific health concerns.

ΔΔΔ

Certain supplements may interact with prescription drugs, over-the-counter medications, or other supplements, leading to adverse effects or reduced effectiveness.

Here is a list of commonly utilized supplements, along with potential drug interactions and recommended precautions to ensure safe usage.

ST. JOHN'S WORT

- Interactions: Can reduce the effectiveness of various medications, including antidepressants, birth control pills, blood thinners, and certain HIV medications.
- Counteraction: Avoid combining St. John's Wort with medications affected by its interactions.

GINKGO BILOBA

- Interactions: May interact with blood thinners, antidepressants, anticonvulsants, and certain medications metabolized by the liver.
- Counteraction: Monitor for signs of bleeding

or changes in medication effectiveness in combination with blood thinners.

GARLIC

- Interactions: Garlic may interact with blood thinners, HIV medications, and medications metabolized by the liver.
- Counteraction: Monitor for signs of bleeding or changes in medication effectiveness in combination with blood thinners.

FISH OIL

- Interactions: Fish oil may interact with blood thinners, antiplatelet drugs, and certain medications for high blood pressure.
- Counteraction: Monitor for signs of bleeding or changes in blood pressure in combination with blood thinners.

VITAMIN D

- Interactions: Vitamin D may interact with certain medications for heart disease, high blood pressure, and kidney disease.
- Counteraction: Monitor for changes in medication effectiveness or calcium levels if taking high doses.

IRON

- Interactions: Iron supplements may interact with certain medications for thyroid disorders, antibiotics, and medications for Parkinson's

disease.
- Counteraction: Take iron supplements at least 2 hours apart from medications to reduce the risk of interactions.

CALCIUM

- Interactions: Calcium supplements may interact with certain antibiotics, thyroid medications, and medications for osteoporosis.
- Counteraction: Take calcium supplements at least 2 hours apart from medications to reduce the risk of interactions.

COENZYME Q10

- Interactions: CoQ10 may interact with blood thinners, blood pressure medications, and certain chemotherapy drugs.
- Counteraction: Monitor for changes in blood pressure or bleeding in combination with blood thinners.

MAGNESIUM

- Interactions: Magnesium supplements may interact with certain antibiotics, diuretics, and medications for heart disease.
- Counteraction: Take magnesium supplements at least 2 hours apart from medications to reduce the risk of interactions.

VITAMIN B12

- Interactions: Vitamin B12 supplements may interact with certain medications for acid reflux, diabetes, and epilepsy.
- Counteraction: Monitor for changes in medication effectiveness in combination with acid-reducing medications.

VITAMIN C

- Interactions: Vitamin C supplements may interact with certain medications for cancer, blood pressure, and cholesterol.
- Counteraction: Monitor for changes in medication effectiveness or side effects in combination with medications.

ZINC

- Interactions: Zinc supplements may interact with certain antibiotics, diuretics, and medications for rheumatoid arthritis.
- Counteraction: Take zinc supplements at least 2 hours apart from medications to reduce the risk of interactions.

TURMERIC

- Interactions: Turmeric supplements may interact with blood thinners, antiplatelet drugs, and certain medications for diabetes.
- Counteraction: Monitor for signs of bleeding or

changes in blood sugar in combination with blood thinners or diabetes medications.

PROBIOTICS

- Interactions: Probiotic supplements may interact with antibiotics, immunosuppressants, and certain medications for digestive disorders.
- Counteraction: Take probiotics at least 2 hours apart from antibiotics to reduce the risk of interactions.

OMEGA-3 FATTY ACIDS

- Interactions: Omega-3 supplements may interact with blood thinners, antiplatelet drugs, and certain medications for high cholesterol.
- Counteraction: Monitor for signs of bleeding or changes in cholesterol levels in combination with blood thinners or cholesterol-lowering medications.

SELENIUM

- Interactions: Selenium supplements may interact with certain medications for thyroid disorders, anticoagulants, and chemotherapy drugs.
- Counteraction: Monitor for changes in medication effectiveness in combination with thyroid medications or anticoagulants.

MELATONIN

- Interactions: Melatonin supplements may interact with certain medications for blood pressure, diabetes, and immunosuppression.
- Counteraction: Monitor for changes in medication effectiveness or side effects in combination with medications, such as sedatives, anticoagulants and diabetes prescriptions to name a few.

SAW PALMETTO

- Interactions: Saw palmetto supplements may interact with certain medications for prostate disorders and hormone therapy.
- Counteraction: Monitor for changes in medication effectiveness in combination with medications for prostate health or hormone therapy.

COLLAGEN

- Interactions: Collagen supplements may interact with certain medications for joint pain, arthritis, and blood disorders.
- Counteraction: Monitor for changes in medication effectiveness or side effects in combination with medications.

GREEN TEA EXTRACT

- Interactions: Green tea extract may interact with certain medications for blood thinning, chemotherapy, and liver function.
- Counteraction: Monitor for changes in medication effectiveness or side effects in combination with

blood thinners or chemotherapy drugs.

This list is not exhaustive, and there may be other supplements with potential interactions. Be sure to read product labels and follow recommended dosage instructions to minimize the risk of adverse effects.

CHAPTER 26: FOOD CONSUMPTION

The regulation of food, water, and personal hygiene products by the FDA (Food and Drug Administration) in the United States has faced criticism for its perceived lack of stringent regulations compared to other countries, such as the United Kingdom.

In the U.S., the FDA's regulations on additives and ingredients in food and personal care products are often considered less stringent than those of the U.K.'s Food Standards Agency (FSA).

Furthermore, concerns have been raised about the potential influence of the pharmaceutical industry on FDA regulations, with allegations of a "revolving door" between industry executives and regulatory positions within the FDA.

This perceived conflict of interest has led to skepticism about the impartiality and effectiveness of FDA oversight.

The UK's food laws, enforced by the FSA, are often praised for stricter regulations on additives, pesticides, and food labeling. The FSA prioritizes consumer safety and transparency, regularly conducting inspections and assessments to ensure compliance with food safety standards.

Both agencies aim to protect public health and safety, but differences in regulatory approaches and enforcement mechanisms may contribute to variations in food safety standards between the two countries.

△△△

While dairy products are regulated, avoiding these products is important for individuals who are lactose intolerant. Lactose intolerance is a common condition in which the body lacks the enzyme lactase needed to break down lactose, the sugar found in milk and dairy products.

Many Americans and people around the world experience symptoms such as bloating, gas, diarrhea, and abdominal discomfort after consuming dairy products due to lactose intolerance.

When lactose goes undigested in the gut, it passes into the large intestine, where it interacts with bacteria. These bacteria ferment lactose, leading to the production of gases such as hydrogen, methane, and carbon dioxide.

For individuals who are lactose intolerant, avoiding dairy products or opting for lactose-free alternatives can help alleviate symptoms and improve digestive comfort.

Non-dairy sources of calcium include fortified plant-based milk alternatives, leafy greens, nuts, and seeds. These can provide essential nutrients without triggering symptoms of lactose intolerance.

△△△

Regarding meat consumption, it's important to focus on lean protein sources and limit intake to promote optimal health.

Eating excessive amounts of meat, known as meat stacking, can overload the digestive system and contribute to various health issues, including digestive discomfort, inflammation, and increased risk of chronic diseases such as heart disease and certain types of cancer.

To maintain a balanced and nutritious diet, include a variety of protein sources in your meals, including lean meats such as poultry (chicken, turkey), fish, and plant-based proteins like beans, lentils, tofu, and tempeh.

Limiting meat consumption to once daily or a few times a week allows the digestive system enough time to properly digest and metabolize protein while promoting diversity in nutrient intake and supporting overall health and well-being.

Protein is vital for the body's growth, repair, and maintenance of tissues, enzymes, hormones, and other essential molecules. It's often referred to as the building block of life, as the body requires it for various physiological functions.

However, for the body to utilize protein effectively, it must undergo proper conversion, which involves several genetic and metabolic processes. Mutations in the lipid metabolism gene group can impact how the body metabolizes and utilizes fats, indirectly affecting protein metabolism.

Lipids play a crucial role in the absorption of fat-soluble vitamins and the formation of cell membranes, which are essential for various cellular functions, including protein synthesis and metabolism.

Similarly, the methylation gene group is involved in regulating gene expression, repairing DNA, and metabolizing certain compounds, including proteins. Methylation plays a role in converting amino acids (the building blocks of protein) into various compounds used by the body.

Red meat and pork take longer to digest due to their higher fat content and denser protein structure. As these meats are broken down, they can produce uric acid as a byproduct, which, if not adequately eliminated, can lead to conditions like gout and other joint issues.

In contrast, lean meats like turkey, chicken, and fish are healthier options as they contain less fat and are easier to digest. It's important to diversify protein intake and mitigate potential health risks associated with animal protein consumption by incorporating plant-based protein sources previously mentioned.

△△△

Reading food labels is essential for maintaining your health, especially when detoxifying your body. Food labels provide crucial information about the ingredients and nutritional content of products, allowing you to make informed choices about what you consume.

By carefully examining food labels, you can avoid products containing harmful additives, preservatives, artificial sweeteners, and other toxins that may undermine your detox efforts and become problematic for your health.

In prioritizing whole, natural foods and avoiding processed products with lengthy ingredient lists and unfamiliar additives, you can support proper function of your body. Making a habit of reading food labels empowers you to take control of your diet and make choices that align with your health goals.

Here's a list of toxic food additives:

- Artificial Sweeteners (e.g., Aspartame, Sucralose): Linked to various health issues, including headaches, digestive problems, and even cancer in some studies. To detox from artificial sweeteners, focus on consuming whole, natural foods and beverages without added sweeteners.

- Monosodium Glutamate (MSG): Known to cause symptoms like headaches, flushing, sweating, and numbness in some individuals. To detox from MSG, opt for homemade meals using fresh ingredients instead of processed foods.

- High Fructose Corn Syrup (HFCS): Associated with obesity, type 2 diabetes, and other metabolic disorders due to its high concentration of fructose. To detox from HFCS, limit consumption of processed foods and beverages and choose whole fruits instead of sugary snacks.

- Artificial Food Dyes (e.g., Red 40, Yellow 5, Blue 1): Linked to behavioral problems in children, allergies, anxiety, and hyperactivity. To detox from artificial food dyes, focus on eating foods with natural colors and avoiding products with added synthetic dyes.

- Sodium Nitrite and Nitrate: Found in processed

meats and linked to an increased risk of cancer, particularly colorectal cancer. To detox from sodium nitrite and nitrate, limit consumption of processed meats and choose nitrate-free options when available.

- Trans Fats (Partially Hydrogenated Oils): Increase the risk of heart disease by raising LDL (bad) cholesterol and lowering HDL (good) cholesterol levels. To detox from trans fats, avoid fried foods, baked goods, and processed snacks containing partially hydrogenated oils.

- Gluten: Can cause digestive issues and inflammation in individuals with gluten sensitivity or celiac disease. To detox from gluten, choose gluten-free grains like quinoa, rice, and buckwheat, and opt for gluten-free versions of packaged foods.

- Dairy: Some people are lactose intolerant or sensitive to dairy proteins, which can cause digestive problems, skin issues, and respiratory symptoms. To detox from dairy, try dairy-free alternatives like almond milk, coconut milk, or soy milk, and avoid products containing milk, cheese, and yogurt.

To detox from these toxic additives, focus on consuming a balanced diet rich in whole, natural foods, including plenty of fruits, vegetables, whole grains, lean proteins, and healthy fats.

Drink plenty of water to help flush toxins from your system, and consider consulting with a healthcare professional for personalized advice.

△△△

A significant portion of the food available in stores today contains genetically modified organisms (GMO) ingredients. These are organisms whose genetic material has been altered using engineering techniques.

This technology allows scientists to introduce specific traits into plants or animals, such as resistance to pests or tolerance to herbicides. One of the most recent and significant advancements in this technology is CRISPR-Cas9.

CRISPR-Cas9 is a gene-editing tool that allows scientists to modify DNA sequences within an organism's genome precisely.

When it comes to identifying organic, conventional, and GMO foods, there are specific codes and labels to look for:

- Organic: Certified organic products will have a label indicating such, often with a certification logo from an accredited organization like the USDA Organic or similar certifying bodies in other countries. The code for organic produce usually begins with the number 9.

- Conventional: Conventional foods are those that are produced using conventional farming methods, which may include the use of synthetic pesticides, fertilizers, and GMOs. These products typically start with the number 4.

- GMO: Genetically modified foods may not always be labeled as such, depending on the regulations in your country. Some regions have voluntary labeling initiatives, but they are not universal. However, some countries require labeling of GMO foods, and the code for GMO produce typically begins with the number 8.

△△△

As for recent developments, CRISPR technology continues to advance rapidly, with ongoing research to improve its precision, efficiency, and applicability across various organisms. Scientists are exploring its potential applications in agriculture, medicine, and other fields.

There is ongoing debate and regulatory scrutiny surrounding the use of CRISPR and other gene-editing technologies, particularly regarding safety, ethical concerns, and potential environmental impacts.

While CRISPR-Cas9 holds potential for various applications, including agriculture, medicine, and biotechnology, there are also several risks and ethical considerations associated with its use:

- Off-target Effects: One of the primary concerns with CRISPR is the potential for off-target effects, where the gene-editing tool may unintentionally modify other parts of the genome, leading to unpredictable consequences. Researchers continuously work to minimize off-target effects through improved design and delivery methods.

- Unknown Long-term Effects: The long-term effects of CRISPR-mediated genetic modifications are not fully understood. Changes made to an organism's genome could have unintended consequences that may not become apparent until much later, posing risks to both the modified organism and its ecosystem.

- Ethical Concerns: The ability to edit the human germline raises ethical questions about the potential for heritable genetic modifications. Concerns also arise about the implications of altering the genetic makeup of future generations, including issues related to consent, equity, and unintended social consequences.

- Unintended Consequences: Introducing genetically modified organisms into the environment could have unintended ecological consequences, such as disrupting ecosystems, affecting biodiversity, or promoting the evolution of resistant pests or pathogens.

- Dual-use Concerns: CRISPR technology could be misused for malicious purposes, such as bioterrorism or the creation of bioengineered pathogens. Safeguards and regulations are needed to prevent the misuse of gene-editing technologies for harmful purposes.

- Regulatory Challenges: The rapid pace of CRISPR research and development has outpaced regulatory frameworks in many countries, leading to challenges in assessing the safety and ethical implications of CRISPR applications and ensuring appropriate oversight.

△△△

Then there's the concept of growing food in labs, often referred to as cellular agriculture or cultured meat. Cellular agriculture involves producing food products such as meat, dairy, and even certain types of produce using cell culture techniques instead of traditional farming methods.

This technology is still in its early stages; however, there are also safety concerns and regulatory challenges associated with lab-grown food.

These include:

- Food Safety: Ensuring the safety of lab-grown food products is a critical consideration. Scientists must develop methods to minimize the risk of contamination and ensure that the final products meet food safety standards and nutritional requirements.

- Regulatory Oversight: Regulatory agencies are grappling with how to classify and regulate lab-grown food products. Due to the novel nature of these products, determining appropriate safety standards, labeling requirements, and oversight mechanisms poses challenges.

- Acceptance: Consumer acceptance of lab-grown foods may be influenced by taste, price, perceived safety, and cultural attitudes toward food production methods. Educating consumers and addressing concerns about the novelty and safety of lab-grown foods will be essential for widespread adoption.

△△△

Another serious concern is vaccines in produce like lettuce, while there has been speculation and research into edible vaccines. Edible vaccines are a theoretical concept where plants are genetically modified to produce antigens from pathogens, effectively turning them into a vehicle for delivering vaccines orally.

Proponents say the idea of edible vaccines presents benefits, such as easier distribution and administration, but there are significant scientific, regulatory, and ethical considerations to address.

These include ensuring the safety, efficacy, and stability of the vaccine, addressing concerns about genetic modification; establishing regulatory frameworks for approval and oversight; and addressing public acceptance and ethical concerns surrounding the use of genetically modified organisms for vaccine production.

These concept present possibilities for addressing various challenges in food production, but more regulatory efforts are needed to realize their potential safely and ethically.

ΔΔΔ

How to eat is another important part of the journey.

RHYTHMIC EATING

Also known as chrono-nutrition, this emphasizes aligning meals with the body's natural circadian rhythms to optimize health and metabolism.

Circadian biology expert Dr. Satchin Panda's research suggests that consuming the majority of calories earlier in the day may support better metabolic health and weight management.

In the morning, aim for a balanced breakfast rich in protein, healthy fats, and complex carbohydrates to kickstart metabolism and provide sustained energy throughout the day.

Options include:

- Lean protein sources such as eggs, Greek yogurt, or tofu
- Whole grain toast or oats for complex carbohydrates
- Nut butter or avocado for healthy fats

For snacks, choose nutrient-dense options like fruits, vegetables, nuts, or seeds to keep energy levels stable between meals.

In the afternoon, focus on a well-rounded lunch containing protein, fiber, and colorful vegetables to support satiety and productivity.

Examples include:

- Grilled chicken or fish with quinoa and roasted vegetables
- Salad with mixed greens, chickpeas, avocado, and olive oil dressing

In the evening, opt for a lighter dinner consisting of lean protein, non-starchy vegetables, and healthy fats to aid digestion and promote restful sleep.

Consider:

- Baked salmon with steamed broccoli and sweet potato
- Stir-fried tofu with mixed vegetables in coconut oil

WHOLE FOOD, PLANT-BASED EATING

Notable herbalist and natural healer Dr. Sebi (Alfredo Darrington Bowman) advocated for a plant-based diet rich in whole foods, emphasizing alkaline-forming foods such as fruits, vegetables, nuts, seeds, and grains. His approach to rhythmic eating focused on consuming predominantly alkaline foods earlier in the day and limiting acidic foods, such as animal proteins and processed foods, later in the evening.

INTERMITTENT FASTING

Kidney specialist and detox expert Dr. Jason Fung, a proponent of intermittent fasting, suggests eating one meal a day and fasting for the rest of the day. This approach, known as OMAD (One Meal A Day), may offer benefits such as weight loss, improved insulin sensitivity, and enhanced autophagy.

When it comes to meat proteins, consider the following options:

- Lean meats: Chicken breast, turkey breast, lean cuts of beef or pork
- Fish: Salmon, tuna, trout, mackerel
- Poultry: Chicken, turkey
- Red meats: Lean cuts of beef or pork, such as sirloin or tenderloin

For plant-based protein sources, explore:

- Legumes: Lentils, chickpeas, black beans, kidney beans
- Tofu and tempeh: Soy-based products rich in protein and nutrients
- Nuts and seeds: Almonds, walnuts, chia seeds, hemp seeds

- Whole grains: Quinoa, brown rice, barley, millet

Mutations in the MTHFR gene can impact folate metabolism and protein breakdown, potentially affecting health outcomes. The two main alleles associated with MTHFR mutations are:

- C677T allele: Individuals with this allele may have reduced enzyme activity, leading to impaired folate metabolism and potentially elevated homocysteine levels.

- A1298C allele: This allele may also affect folate metabolism, although the impact may be less pronounced than that of the C677T allele.

Elevated homocysteine levels can indicate may increase the risk of cardiovascular disease. Homocysteine, commonly found in meat protein, needs to be broken down into methionine, an essential amino acid and key building block for proteins in the body.

Too many undigested proteins can convert into fats and sugars, leading to weight gain, insulin resistance, and metabolic imbalances.

Folate must be converted to 5-MTHF, it's active form and plays a significant role in supporting mitochondrial function and overall cellular health.

The mitochondria is the brain and powerhouse of every cell. Lack of 5-MTHF can contribute to a range of health problems, including neurodegenrative diseases, metabolic disorders and aging-related conditions.

The body requires an adequate intake of protein to support various physiological functions, including:

- Muscle growth and repair: Protein provides the essential amino acids necessary for building and repairing muscle tissue, especially after exercise or injury.

- Enzyme and hormone production: Many enzymes and hormones are made up of proteins, which play crucial roles in metabolic processes, digestion, and signaling within the body.

- Immune function: Antibodies, which help fight infections and pathogens, are proteins produced by the immune system in response to foreign invaders.

- Transport and storage: Proteins transport nutrients, oxygen, and waste products throughout the body and can store essential molecules such as iron and oxygen in tissues and cells.

- Structural support: Proteins form the structural components of cells, tissues, and organs, providing strength and stability to the body's framework.

- Energy production: While carbohydrates and fats are the body's primary sources of energy, protein can be converted into glucose through a process called gluconeogenesis during periods of fasting or low carbohydrate intake. Protein is not typically used as a primary energy source under normal conditions.

Protein plays a vital role in maintaining health and well-being, and ensuring an adequate and diversified intake through dietary sources is essential for optimal function and performance.

CHAPTER 27: PROPER HYDRATION

The amount of water a person should consume daily varies depending on age, weight, activity level, climate, and overall health. However, the general guideline for water consumption is around eight glasses of water per day, roughly two liters or half a gallon. Some experts suggest even more, especially for individuals living in hot climates or engaging in vigorous physical activity.

Water is crucial for various physiological functions in the body. It plays a vital role in converting food into energy through the process of metabolism. Additionally, water helps transport nutrients to cells and remove waste products from the body. It aids in digestion by lubricating the digestive tract and facilitating the absorption of nutrients.

Approximately 60% of the human body is composed of water. Here's a breakdown of water distribution by organs and systems:

- Brain and Heart: Both the brain and heart are composed of about 73% water.
  - Lungs: Approximately 83% of the lungs consist of water, which is crucial for maintaining proper

respiratory function.

- Muscles and Kidneys: Muscles are composed of around 79% water, while the kidneys, responsible for filtering waste from the blood, contain about 79-83% water.

- Skin: The skin, the body's largest organ, contains about 64% water, which helps maintain skin elasticity and hydration.

- Blood: Blood is about 83% water and serves as the medium for transporting oxygen, nutrients, and hormones throughout the body.

Given the vital role of water in the body's overall function and health, staying adequately hydrated is essential for maintaining optimal physiological processes. It's important to listen to your body's cues for thirst and drink water regularly throughout the day to ensure proper hydration.

Proper hydration is essential for overall health, and alkaline water has gained attention for its potential benefits in supporting hydration and promoting a more alkaline environment in the body.

Alkaline water has a higher pH level than regular tap water, which may help neutralize acidity in the body and offer additional health benefits. Alkaline water's smaller molecular size allows it to penetrate cells more readily, facilitating better hydration and oxygenation.

Other hydration options I recommend include:

- Hydrogen water: Hydrogen water is water that has been infused with molecular hydrogen (H_2) gas. Proponents claim that hydrogen water possesses antioxidant properties and may offer health benefits such as reducing inflammation, improving athletic performance, and protecting against oxidative stress.

- Reverse osmosis water: Reverse osmosis (RO) water is produced by a filtration process that removes impurities, including minerals, chemicals, and contaminants, from water by applying pressure to force it through a semi-permeable membrane. This process results in highly purified water with a low mineral content, making it suitable for various applications, including drinking water and industrial processes.

- Mineral water: Mineral water is sourced from natural springs or wells and contains various minerals and trace elements, such as calcium, magnesium, and potassium, which are dissolved in the surrounding rocks and soil. Mineral water is often marketed for its perceived health benefits and may be consumed for hydration and mineral supplementation.

- Distilled water: Distilled water is produced by boiling water to create steam, which is then condensed back into liquid form. This process effectively removes impurities, minerals, and contaminants from the water, resulting in a highly purified product. Due to its purity, distilled water is commonly used in laboratory experiments, medical procedures, and automotive batteries.

Tap water often contains additives like chlorine and fluoride, which some researchers argue may increase the size of water molecules and impact their ability to hydrate cells effectively. Mutations or deletions within the genetic code may also hinder the body's conversion of regular H2O into structured water (H3O2), which is more readily absorbed by cells.

If you're on a budget, you can alkalize water at home using natural ingredients such as Himalayan pink salt or Celtic Sea salt. These unrefined salts contain minerals and trace elements that can help raise the pH level of water and impart additional health benefits.

Adding a small pinch of either type of salt to a glass of water can create alkalized water that offers health benefits, such as improved digestion and increased energy levels. Another popular way to alkalize water is to squeeze a lemon into it. Let it marinate overnight for best results and then drink.

△△△

Juicing has also become a trend in the health and wellness community, offering a convenient way to boost nutrient intake and support overall well-being. From cold-pressed to centrifugal juicing methods, there are various approaches to extracting the liquid goodness from fruits and vegetables.

Let's go through the benefits of juicing, different juicing methods, the best fruits and vegetables to juice, juicing combinations for various health ailments, and the fascinating world of structured water, known as H3O2.

Juicing offers a plethora of benefits for both body and mind. Firstly, it provides a concentrated source of essential vitamins, minerals, and antioxidants vital for optimal health. By extracting the liquid essence of fruits and vegetables, juicing makes these nutrients more readily available for absorption, supporting overall vitality and immune function.

Additionally, juicing can aid in hydration, as fresh juices

provide a hydrating boost while delivering essential nutrients to cells. Advocates of juicing assert that it aids in clearing mucus from the body, where parasites, Candida, and fungus thrive. By eliminating excess mucus through juicing, the body can expel these harmful organisms and promote overall health.

There are several juicing methods to choose from, each with its unique advantages:

- Cold-pressed juicing: Involves using a hydraulic press to extract juice from produce without generating heat, preserving the nutrients and enzymes present in the fruits and vegetables.

- Centrifugal juicing: Utilizes high-speed spinning to separate the juice from the pulp, offering a quick and convenient option for juicing.

- Masticating juicing: Uses a slow grinding motion to extract juice, minimizing heat exposure and oxidation.

- Blending: Involves blending whole fruits and vegetables into a smoothie-like consistency, retaining the fiber content of the produce.

When it comes to juicing, variety is key. Some of the best fruits and vegetables to juice include:

- Fruits: Apples, oranges, berries (blueberries, strawberries, and raspberries), pineapple, kiwi, watermelon.

- Vegetables: Leafy greens (kale, spinach, and Swiss chard), cucumbers, celery, carrots, beets, and ginger.

Juicing can be tailored to address specific health concerns by combining fruits and vegetables rich in nutrients that target particular ailments.

Here are ten juicing combinations and the health issues they may address:

- Immune Booster: Kale, spinach, ginger, lemon, and apple. Helps strengthen the immune system and fight off infections.

- Digestive Health: Celery, cucumber, ginger, lemon, and mint. Supports digestion and relieves bloating.

- Anti-Inflammatory: Turmeric, pineapple, ginger, and carrot. Reduces inflammation and alleviates pain.

- Detoxification: Beet, carrot, apple, lemon, and ginger. Supports liver detoxification and removes toxins from the body.

- Skin Health: Carrot, orange, cucumber, and spinach. Nourishes the skin and promotes a healthy complexion.

- Energy Booster: Spinach, kale, celery, cucumber, and apple. Provides a natural energy boost and improves vitality.

- Stress Relief: Blueberries, strawberries, kale, and ginger. Helps reduce stress and promotes relaxation.

- Bone Health: Broccoli, kale, orange, and lemon. Rich in calcium and vitamin C for strong bones.

- Heart Health: Beet, carrot, apple, and ginger. Supports cardiovascular health and lowers blood pressure.

- Weight Loss: Grapefruit, cucumber, celery, and mint. Aids in weight management and promotes fat loss.

When juicing for specific health concerns, it's essential to use fresh, organic produce and adjust the quantities to suit your taste preferences and individual needs. Experiment with different combinations and monitor how your body responds to find your optimal juicing regimen.

It is important to point out how juicing aligns seamlessly with the concept of structured water, also known as H3O2. Structured water is a unique molecular arrangement that enhances its hydrating properties and bioavailability.

While scientific research on structured water is still emerging, proponents suggest that it may offer benefits such as improved cellular hydration, detoxification, and antioxidant activity.

Natural springs, ionization devices, and certain fruits and vegetables serve as sources of structured water, providing essential hydration and supporting overall well-being. By incorporating fresh juices into our diet, we not only nourish our bodies with vital nutrients but also contribute to optimal hydration and cellular health.

△△△

Infused waters and teas can add variety to your daily required water consumption and support the body's natural detoxification processes. Experiment with different combinations and adjust the flavors to suit your taste preferences.

Here are a few examples:

- Lemon and Mint Infused Water: Lemon helps to alkalize the body and aid digestion, while mint adds a refreshing flavor and can soothe the stomach.

- Cucumber and Mint Infused Water: Cucumber is hydrating and contains antioxidants, while mint adds a refreshing taste and aids digestion.

- Ginger and Lemon Infused Water: Ginger is known for its anti-inflammatory properties and can help with digestion, while lemon adds a citrusy flavor and helps detoxify the body.

- Strawberry and Basil Infused Water: Strawberries are rich in antioxidants and vitamin C, while basil adds a hint of sweetness and contains anti-inflammatory properties.

- Watermelon and Rosemary Infused Water: Watermelon is hydrating and contains lycopene, while rosemary adds a unique flavor and has antioxidant properties.

- Blueberry and Lavender Infused Water: Blueberries are packed with antioxidants, while lavender adds a floral aroma and can help promote relaxation.

- Orange and Thyme Infused Water: Oranges are high in vitamin C and antioxidants, while thyme adds a savory flavor and contains antibacterial properties.

These teas are commonly used for detoxification:

- Green Tea: Contains antioxidants called catechins,

which may support liver health and boost metabolism.

- Dandelion Tea: Acts as a natural diuretic, promoting detoxification by increasing urine production and supporting liver function.

- Ginger Tea: Helps stimulate digestion, alleviates nausea, and has anti-inflammatory properties that support detoxification.

- Peppermint Tea: Soothes the digestive tract, reduces bloating, and may support liver and gallbladder function.

- Turmeric Tea: Contains curcumin, a potent antioxidant with anti-inflammatory properties that may support detoxification and liver health.

- Nettle Tea: Acts as a diuretic and may help cleanse the urinary tract, support kidney function, and alleviate allergies.

- Milk Thistle Tea: Contains silymarin, a compound known for its liver-protective properties, making it beneficial for detoxification.

- Lemon Detox Tea: Combines lemon juice with hot water, which may stimulate digestion, support liver function, and promote hydration.

- Hibiscus Tea: Rich in antioxidants and vitamin C, hibiscus tea may support liver health, reduce oxidative stress, and promote overall detoxification.

- Rooibos Tea: Naturally caffeine-free, rooibos tea is rich in antioxidants and may support liver health, digestion, and overall well-being.

Infused water or teas can be used as part of a balanced diet and healthy lifestyle to support the body's natural detoxification processes.

CHAPTER 28: EYE DISEASE, DETOX & IRIDOLOGY

Eye diseases and disorders impact millions of individuals worldwide, affecting their quality of life and potentially leading to vision impairment or blindness.

According to the World Health Organization, over 2 billion people have vision impairment or blindness, with conditions ranging from cataracts and glaucoma to age-related macular degeneration and diabetic retinopathy.

These conditions can arise from a variety of causes, including genetics, age, environmental factors, and systemic diseases like diabetes.

Exposure to heavy metals, parasites, such as Demodex mites, and liver or kidney disease can also contribute to eye problems. Treatments vary from holistic approaches like castor oil massages to allopathic interventions, such as medications and surgical procedures.

Top eye conditions include:

- Cataracts: Characterized by clouding of the lens, leading to blurred vision and eventual blindness if left untreated. It's one of the leading causes of blindness globally.

- Glaucoma: A group of eye conditions that damage the optic nerve, often due to increased pressure in the eye. It can result in vision loss and blindness.

- Age-related macular degeneration (AMD): This affects the macula, the central part of the retina, leading to a loss of central vision. It's a common cause of vision impairment in older adults.

- Diabetic retinopathy: Caused by damage to the blood vessels in the retina due to diabetes. It can lead to vision loss and blindness if not managed properly.

- Refractive errors: Include myopia (nearsightedness), hyperopia (farsightedness), astigmatism, and presbyopia (age-related difficulty focusing close up).

These eye diseases and disorders can have various causes, including:

- Genetics: Many eye conditions have a genetic component, making individuals more susceptible if there's a family history.

- Age: Some conditions, like cataracts and AMD, become more common with age.

- Environmental factors: Exposure to UV radiation, pollution, and certain chemicals can increase the risk of developing eye diseases.

- Lifestyle factors: Poor diet, smoking, and lack of exercise can contribute to the development of eye conditions.

- Systemic diseases: Conditions like diabetes,

hypertension, and autoimmune diseases can affect the eyes.

- Heavy metal toxicity: Exposure to heavy metals like lead, mercury, and arsenic can damage the eyes and contribute to various eye disorders.

- Parasites: Certain parasites, such as Toxoplasma gondii and Onchocerca volvulus, can infect the eyes and cause conditions like toxoplasmosis and river blindness.

- Demodex: These microscopic mites can infest the eyelashes and hair follicles, leading to blepharitis and other eye problems.

- Liver and kidney disease: Dysfunction in these organs can manifest in the eyes as yellowing (jaundice) or changes in vision due to metabolic imbalances.

ΔΔΔ

The eyes are the window to the soul, but they can also be the first resource to assess a person's health status and potential predispositions to certain diseases or imbalances within the body.

Practitioners of iridology believe that various patterns, colors, and markings in the iris can provide insights into an individual's overall health and well-being.

The underlying theory of iridology is that different areas of the iris correspond to specific organs and systems in the body. By closely examining these patterns and markings, iridologists say they can identify areas of weakness, inflammation, or toxicity within the body.

Iridologists use specialized equipment such as a magnifying glass or camera to observe the iris in detail. They also use charts or maps that correlate specific areas of the iris with corresponding organs or body systems.

Based on their observations, iridologists may make recommendations for lifestyle changes, dietary modifications, or detoxification protocols to help restore balance and improve health.

Some individuals may find iridology valuable as a complementary or alternative approach to health assessment. Its use as a diagnostic tool should be approached with caution, however.

△△△

Remedies for eye diseases and disorders vary depending on the condition and its severity. One that has been very effective for me is castor oil. It can be effective in promoting eye healing for several reasons:

- Anti-inflammatory properties: Castor oil contains ricinoleic acid, which has known anti-inflammatory properties. When applied to the eyelids, castor oil can help reduce inflammation, redness, and irritation, relieving conditions such as dry eyes and blepharitis.

- Moisturizing and lubricating: Castor oil is a rich source of fatty acids, which help moisturize and lubricate the eyes. It can be particularly beneficial for individuals suffering from dry eye syndrome, as it helps alleviate dryness and discomfort by providing a protective layer over the ocular surface.

- Antimicrobial effects: Some research suggests that castor oil may possess antimicrobial properties, which can help prevent bacterial and fungal infections on the eyelids and around the eyes. It can benefit individuals with conditions like blepharitis, where microbial overgrowth can contribute to inflammation and irritation.

- Promotes eyelash growth: Castor oil is also believed to promote eyelash growth and thickness. Applying castor oil to the eyelashes can help strengthen the hair follicles and stimulate growth, resulting in longer, fuller lashes.

While more research is needed to fully understand the mechanisms behind castor oil's effectiveness in eye healing, the many benefits make it a popular choice for eye health and healing.

It's essential to use castor oil carefully and consult with a healthcare professional, especially if you have pre-existing eye conditions or allergies.

Here are some other supplements and nutrients that support eye health and potentially improve eyesight:

- Vitamin A: Essential for maintaining good vision, particularly in low-light conditions. Sources include liver, carrots, sweet potatoes, spinach, and kale.

- Vitamin C: An antioxidant that helps protect the eyes from damage caused by free radicals. Found in citrus fruits, strawberries, bell peppers, and broccoli.

- Vitamin E: Another antioxidant that may reduce the risk of cataracts and age-related macular degeneration. Sources include nuts, seeds, vegetable oils, and leafy greens.

- Lutein and Zeaxanthin: Carotenoids that accumulate in the retina and help filter harmful blue light. Found in spinach, kale, broccoli, and egg yolks.

- Omega-3 fatty acids: Essential for maintaining retinal health and reducing the risk of dry eyes and macular degeneration. Sources include fatty fish like salmon, mackerel, and sardines, as well as flaxseeds, chia seeds, and walnuts.

- Zinc: Important for the metabolism of vitamin A and the maintenance of healthy retinas. Found in meat, shellfish, legumes, nuts, and seeds.

- Bioflavonoids: Plant compounds with antioxidant properties that may help protect the eyes from damage. Sources include citrus fruits, berries, onions, and tea.

- Bilberry: Contains anthocyanins, which may improve blood flow to the eyes and help with night vision. Available as a supplement or in the form of fresh or dried berries.

- Astaxanthin: A powerful antioxidant that may help reduce eye fatigue and improve visual acuity. Found in seafood like salmon, shrimp, and krill, as well as in supplement form.

- Ginkgo biloba: May improve blood flow to the eyes and protect against age-related eye diseases. Available as a supplement.

While these supplements and nutrients may support overall eye health, it's essential to obtain them as part of a balanced diet rather than relying solely on supplements.

△△△

Biotissue is a regenerative ocular health company that specializes in developing and manufacturing regenerative and therapeutic tissue-based products for various medical applications, particularly in ophthalmology.

Here are two of their products:

- Cliradex: A product line that focuses on eyelid and eyelash hygiene. It contains natural ingredients, including 4-Terpineol, derived from tea tree oil, which has been shown to have antimicrobial properties. Cliradex products are used for the management of conditions such as blepharitis, Demodex infestation (demodicosis), and dry eye syndrome by promoting clean and healthy eyelids.

- Prokera: This is a therapeutic device used for the management of various ocular surface diseases and conditions. It consists of a piece of amniotic membrane tissue preserved in a cryopreservation process. When placed on the eye, Prokera acts as a biologic bandage, providing a protective barrier and delivering healing factors to the ocular surface. It is commonly used for treating conditions such as corneal abrasions, chemical burns, and persistent epithelial defects.

Allopathic treatments for eye disease may include:

- Medications: Eye drops, oral medications, or injections to manage symptoms or slow the progression of certain conditions.

- Surgery: Procedures like cataract surgery, laser therapy for glaucoma, or injections for AMD.

CHAPTER 29: LUNG DETOX

Lung disorders affect millions of people worldwide, with various factors such as environmental pollutants, genetic predispositions, and lifestyle habits contributing to their prevalence.

Understanding the body's cascaded inflammation response is crucial in comprehending how genetic factors influence lung function and susceptibility to respiratory diseases. It's a step-by-step reaction initiated by the immune system respond to infections and irritants, which lead to inflammation in the respiratory tract and potential lung damage.

Despite the complexity of lung disorders, effective detoxification methods, including holistic approaches like lifestyle modifications and nutrition, as well as allopathic treatments such as medications and surgery, can help individuals manage symptoms and improve lung health.

By prioritizing lung detoxification and seeking personalized guidance from healthcare professionals, individuals can take proactive steps toward maintaining respiratory well-being and enjoying a healthier life.

Let's explore lung disorders, genetic influences, the body's inflammation response, and effective detoxification methods, including the use of proteolytic enzymes as an anti-inflammatory option.

Here's an overview of some common lung disorders:

- Asthma: Characterized by inflammation and narrowing of the airways, resulting in wheezing, coughing, and shortness of breath, often triggered by allergens or irritants.

- Chronic obstructive pulmonary disease (COPD): A progressive lung disease that includes emphysema and chronic bronchitis, leading to airflow limitation and difficulty breathing.

- Bronchitis: Inflammation of the bronchial tubes, typically caused by viral or bacterial infections, resulting in coughing, mucus production, and chest discomfort.

- Pneumonia: An infection of the lung tissue caused by bacteria, viruses, or fungi, leading to symptoms such as fever, cough, chest pain, and difficulty breathing.

- Lung cancer: Abnormal cell growth in the lungs, often associated with smoking but can also occur in non-smokers, leading to symptoms such as coughing, chest pain, and weight loss.

- Tuberculosis (TB): A bacterial infection caused by Mycobacterium tuberculosis, primarily affecting the lungs but can spread to other organs, causing symptoms such as coughing, fever, and night sweats.

- Pulmonary fibrosis: Scarring of lung tissue, leading to stiffness and reduced lung function, often of unknown cause but may be associated with environmental exposures or autoimmune diseases.

- Emphysema: Destruction of lung tissue, particularly the alveoli, resulting in reduced elasticity and airflow limitation, commonly associated with smoking.

- Cystic fibrosis: A genetic disorder affecting the lungs and other organs, characterized by thick, sticky mucus production, leading to recurrent infections and respiratory complications.

- Pulmonary hypertension: High blood pressure in the arteries of the lungs, causing symptoms such as shortness of breath, fatigue, and chest pain. Often associated with underlying conditions such as heart or lung disease.

Genetic factors play a significant role in determining lung function and susceptibility to respiratory diseases. Several gene groups are involved in respiratory health, including those responsible for:

- Lung development and structure: Genes involved in lung development during fetal development and maintenance of lung structure throughout life.

- Metabolism of toxins and pollutants: Genes encoding enzymes involved in detoxifying environmental pollutants and toxins that can damage lung tissue.

The body's inflammation response involves a series of steps initiated by the immune system in response to infections and irritants in the respiratory tract.

Here's a breakdown of this process:

- Recognition of the threat: When harmful pathogens or irritants enter the respiratory tract, immune cells such as macrophages and dendritic cells recognize them as foreign invaders.

- Activation of immune cells: Upon recognition, immune cells release signaling molecules called cytokines, which trigger the activation and recruitment of additional immune cells to the site of infection or irritation.

- Inflammatory response: Cytokines stimulate the dilation of blood vessels in the affected area, increasing blood flow and allowing immune cells to reach the site more efficiently. This results in redness, swelling, and heat, which are characteristic of inflammation.

- Phagocytosis: Immune cells, particularly neutrophils and macrophages, engulf and destroy pathogens through a process called phagocytosis. Phagocytosis helps to eliminate the threat and prevent further infection.

- Tissue repair and resolution: Once the threat is neutralized, anti-inflammatory signals are released to dampen the immune response and promote tissue repair. Fibroblasts produce collagen to repair damaged tissue, and the inflammatory process gradually subsides.

△△△

In cases of chronic inflammation or persistent exposure to irritants, this cascaded inflammation response can become dysregulated, leading to prolonged tissue damage and exacerbation of respiratory conditions such as asthma, COPD, and pulmonary fibrosis. Understanding and modulating this inflammatory response is crucial for managing and treating lung disorders effectively.

Here are some holistic ways to achieve relief:

PROTEOLYTIC ENZYMES

Bromelain, papain, and serrapeptase, have gained attention for their anti-inflammatory and detoxifying properties. These enzymes break down proteins in the body, reducing inflammation and promoting tissue repair. When used as a supplement, proteolytic enzymes may help alleviate lung inflammation and support detoxification processes.

MULLEIN LEAF

This has a long history of use in traditional medicine for respiratory health and lung detoxification. It contains various bioactive compounds, including saponins, mucilage, flavonoids, and phenolic acids, which contribute to its therapeutic properties.

Here are some of the benefits of mullein leaf and its various forms and uses for lung detox:

- Expectorant properties: Mullein leaf is known for its expectorant properties, meaning it helps promote the expulsion of mucus from the respiratory tract. These properties make it beneficial for conditions such as bronchitis, asthma, and coughs associated with excess mucus production.

- Anti-inflammatory effects: Mullein leaf exhibits anti-inflammatory properties, which can help reduce inflammation in the airways and ease symptoms of respiratory conditions such as asthma and bronchitis.

- Antibacterial and antiviral activity: Mullein leaf has demonstrated antibacterial and antiviral activity against various pathogens, making it useful for supporting the immune system and fighting respiratory infections.

- Demulcent action: The mucilage content in mullein leaf provides a soothing and protective coating to irritated mucous membranes in the respiratory tract, helping to alleviate dryness, irritation, and cough.

- Lung detoxification: Mullein leaf is believed to support lung detoxification by helping to clear congestion, remove toxins, and support overall respiratory health. It can be used as part of a holistic approach to lung detoxification, along with other supportive measures such as hydration, deep breathing exercises, and dietary changes.

Mullein leaf can be utilized in various forms for lung detoxification, including:

- Tea: Mullein leaf tea is a popular and convenient way to reap its respiratory benefits. Simply steep dried mullein leaves in hot water for 10-15 minutes, strain, and drink. You can add honey or lemon for flavor if desired.

- Tincture: Mullein leaf tincture is made by

extracting the bioactive compounds from the leaves using alcohol or glycerin. It can be taken orally by adding a few drops to water or juice.

- Inhalation: Inhaling steam infused with mullein leaf can help moisten and soothe the respiratory passages, making it easier to expel mucus and alleviate congestion. You can do this by adding dried mullein leaves to hot water and inhaling the steam or by using a steam inhaler.

- Capsules or tablets: Mullein leaf supplements are available in capsule or tablet form for convenient consumption and can be taken orally as directed by the manufacturer.

PEPPERMINT ESSENTIAL OIL

Another option for the lungs is peppermint essential oil, renowned for opening up the respiratory passages and promoting easier breathing.

It contains a compound called menthol, which has a cooling and soothing effect on the nasal passages and airways.

When inhaled, peppermint oil can help alleviate symptoms of congestion, sinusitis, and respiratory conditions such as asthma and bronchitis by reducing inflammation and promoting airway relaxation.

In addition to its respiratory benefits, peppermint essential oil offers a range of other therapeutic properties:

- Digestive support: Peppermint oil has been traditionally used to relieve digestive issues such as indigestion, bloating, and gas. It helps relax the muscles of the digestive tract, easing discomfort and promoting healthy digestion.

- Pain relief: The menthol content in peppermint oil provides a cooling sensation that can help alleviate muscle aches, headaches, and tension. It is commonly used in topical preparations for pain relief and massage therapy.

- Mental clarity and alertness: The invigorating aroma of peppermint oil is known to stimulate the mind, enhance focus, and improve mental clarity. It can be diffused in the air or applied topically to the temples and wrists for an energy boost and heightened concentration.

- Antimicrobial properties: Peppermint oil exhibits antimicrobial activity against various pathogens, including bacteria, viruses, and fungi. It can be used as a natural disinfectant for cleaning surfaces or as an ingredient in homemade cleaning products.

Top essential oil companies known for their high-quality products include:

- doTERRA: Known for their Certified Pure Therapeutic Grade (CPTG) essential oils, doTERRA sources their oils from reputable growers around the world and rigorously tests them for purity and potency.

- Young Living: Young Living offers a wide range of essential oils, including peppermint oil, which are produced through their Seed to Seal® quality assurance process. This process ensures that their oils are responsibly sourced, carefully distilled, and free from contaminants.

- Plant Therapy: Plant Therapy is committed to providing affordable, high-quality essential oils that are free from additives and adulterants. They offer third-party testing results for transparency and assurance of product quality.

- Rocky Mountain Oils: Rocky Mountain Oils offers a diverse selection of pure essential oils, including peppermint oil, sourced from ethical suppliers and tested for purity and potency.

When purchasing essential oils, choosing reputable companies that prioritize quality, transparency, and sustainability in their sourcing and production practices is essential.

△△△

Here are some other approaches to lung detoxification and respiratory health through lifestyle modifications, nutrition, and natural therapies:

- Quit smoking/vaping/hookah: Smoking, regardless of the substance, is one of the leading causes of lung damage and respiratory diseases. Quitting smoking is crucial for lung health and detoxification.

- Air purification: Use air purifiers to remove pollutants and allergens from indoor air, creating a cleaner breathing environment.

- Deep breathing exercises: Practice deep breathing techniques such as diaphragmatic breathing to improve lung function and oxygenation.

- Herbal remedies: Certain herbs, like mullein,

thyme, and eucalyptus, have expectorant and anti-inflammatory properties that can support lung health.

- Steam inhalation: Inhaling steam with essential oils like eucalyptus or peppermint can help clear congestion and soothe irritated airways.

- Stay hydrated: Drink plenty of water to keep mucus thin and promote effective coughing to expel toxins from the lungs.

- Exercise regularly: Engage in regular physical activity to strengthen respiratory muscles, improve lung capacity, and enhance overall cardiovascular health.

- Maintain a healthy diet: Eat a balanced diet rich in fruits, vegetables, whole grains, and lean proteins to provide essential nutrients that support lung function and detoxification.

In addition to holistic approaches, allopathic treatments may be necessary to manage and treat lung disorders, especially in more severe cases.

These include:

- Medications: Bronchodilators, corticosteroids, antibiotics, and other medications may be prescribed to manage symptoms and control inflammation.

- Oxygen therapy: Supplemental oxygen therapy may be recommended for individuals with low blood oxygen levels due to lung disease.

- Pulmonary rehabilitation: Pulmonary rehabilitation programs incorporate exercise, education, and lifestyle modifications to improve lung function and quality of life.

- Surgery: In some cases, surgical interventions such as lung resection or lung transplant may be necessary to treat advanced lung diseases like lung cancer or emphysema.

By understanding the various lung disorders, genetic influences, the body's inflammation response, and effective detoxification methods, individuals can take proactive steps to support lung function and overall well-being.

CHAPTER 30: FASTING

Fasting has gained popularity for its potential health benefits, ranging from weight loss to improved metabolic health and longevity. With various fasting methods available, it's essential to understand the different types, their benefits, precautions, and how to implement them safely.

I don't recommend water fasting, but I've included information about it. I am a strong proponent of juice fasting because while you flush, you restore mineral content and electrolytes with fruit.

Here are the various ways you can fast:

INTERMITTENT FASTING

This involves alternating between periods of eating and fasting. Popular methods include the 16:8 method (fasting for 16 hours and eating within an 8-hour window), alternate-day fasting, and the 5:2 method (eating normally for five days and restricting calories for two non-consecutive days).

Benefits include:

- Weight loss: Intermittent fasting can lead to

reduced calorie intake and increased fat burning, resulting in weight loss.

- Improved metabolic health: It may lower insulin levels, improve insulin sensitivity, and reduce the risk of type 2 diabetes.

- Cellular repair: Fasting triggers cellular repair processes, including autophagy, where cells remove dysfunctional components.

- Longevity: Some studies suggest that intermittent fasting may promote longevity by enhancing cellular health and reducing inflammation.

Precautions to keep in mind:

- Nutrient deficiencies: Fasting periods may lead to inadequate intake of essential nutrients, so it's crucial to consume nutrient-dense foods during eating windows.

- Unsuitability for certain individuals: Intermittent fasting may not be suitable for everyone, especially those with certain medical conditions or eating disorders. Consult a healthcare professional before starting.

How-to:

- Choose a fasting method that suits your lifestyle and preferences.

- Start gradually and listen to your body's hunger cues.

- Stay hydrated during fasting periods and consume balanced meals during eating windows.

JUICE FASTING

This entails consuming only fresh fruit and vegetable juices for a specified period, ranging from a few days to a few weeks.

Benefits include:

- Detoxification: Juice fasting may promote detoxification by increasing the intake of antioxidants and supporting liver function.

- Nutrient intake: It provides a concentrated source of vitamins, minerals, and phytonutrients from fruits and vegetables.

- Potential weight loss: Juice fasting can lead to calorie restriction and weight loss, particularly in the short term.

Precautions to keep in mind:

- Nutrient imbalances: Juice fasting may lack essential nutrients, such as protein and fat, leading to nutrient imbalances and deficiencies.

- Blood sugar spikes: Pure fruit juices, in particular, can cause spikes in blood sugar levels due to their high sugar content. Choose vegetable-based juices or dilute fruit juices with water.

- Unsuitability for certain individuals: Individuals with diabetes or insulin resistance should approach juice fasting with caution due to its impact on blood sugar levels.

How-to:

- Use a variety of fruits and vegetables to create

nutrient-dense juices.

- Consider incorporating protein and healthy fats into your juice recipes, such as adding nut milk or avocado.

- Monitor blood sugar levels regularly, especially if you have diabetes or insulin resistance, and adjust juice recipes accordingly.

WATER FASTING

You only consume water for a specified period, ranging from 24 hours to several days. I highly recommend completing a juice fast before doing a water fast.

Benefits include:

- Cellular repair: Water fasting promotes autophagy and cellular repair, potentially enhancing overall health and longevity.

- Weight loss: It can lead to rapid weight loss by depleting glycogen stores and burning fat for energy.

- Improved insulin sensitivity: Water fasting may improve insulin sensitivity and reduce the risk of insulin resistance.

Precautions to keep in mind:

- Dehydration: Without proper hydration, water fasting can lead to dehydration, electrolyte imbalances, weakness, and dizziness.

- Monitoring: It's essential to monitor electrolyte levels and physical symptoms closely during water fasting.

- Not suitable for everyone: Individuals with certain medical conditions, such as kidney problems or electrolyte imbalances, should avoid water fasting.

How-to:

- Prepare your body by gradually reducing food intake before starting a water fast.
- Drink plenty of water throughout the fasting period to stay hydrated.
- Break the fast gradually with small, easily digestible meals.

ALTERNATE-DAY FASTING

This involves alternating between days of eating normally and fasting. On fasting days, individuals may consume very few calories or none at all.

Benefits include:

- Weight loss: Alternate-day fasting can lead to calorie restriction and increased fat burning, resulting in weight loss.
- Improved heart health: It may lower risk factors for heart disease, such as blood pressure, cholesterol levels, and inflammation.
- Reduced chronic disease risk: Some studies suggest that alternate-day fasting may reduce the risk of chronic diseases, including type 2 diabetes and cancer.

Precautions to keep in mind:

- Overeating: There's a risk of overeating on non-fasting days, which can negate the benefits of fasting. Practice portion control and mindful eating.

- Nutrient intake: Ensure adequate nutrient intake on eating days to prevent nutrient deficiencies.

- Not suitable for everyone: Alternate-day fasting may not be suitable for individuals with certain medical conditions or those prone to disordered eating patterns.

How-to:

- Start with a modified approach, such as reducing calorie intake on fasting days rather than complete fasting.

- Plan balanced meals for eating days to ensure adequate nutrient intake.

- Monitor hunger cues and adjust fasting protocols as needed to maintain adherence.

TIME-RESTRICTED EATING

This involves limiting food intake to a specific window each day, such as eating within a 6- to 8-hour period and fasting for the remaining hours.

Benefits include:

- Weight management: Time-restricted feeding can help regulate appetite, reduce calorie intake, and promote weight loss.

- Improved digestion: It allows the digestive

system to rest during fasting periods, potentially improving digestion and gut health.

- Enhanced metabolic health: Time-restricted feeding may improve insulin sensitivity, blood sugar levels, and lipid profiles.

Precautions to keep in mind:

- Overeating: There's a risk of overeating during the eating window, particularly if meals are not balanced or if individuals have a history of overeating.

- Timing: It's essential to choose a fasting window that aligns with your circadian rhythm and lifestyle to optimize results.

- Individual variability: The effectiveness of time-restricted feeding may vary among individuals, so it's important to experiment and find what works best for you.

How-to:

- Start with a conservative fasting window, such as 12 hours, and gradually increase the fasting duration as tolerated.

- Plan balanced meals that provide essential nutrients and adequate calories within the eating window.

- Pay attention to hunger signals and adjust the fasting window accordingly to ensure sustainability.

Fasting can offer numerous health benefits when done correctly and with caution. It's essential to approach fasting with mindfulness, listening to your body's cues, and seeking medical advice, if necessary.

CHAPTER 31: SELF-ASSESSMENT & MEDICAL TESTING

In the pursuit of optimal health and well-being, embarking on a detox journey has become increasingly popular. Detoxification programs aim to rid the body of toxins, boost energy levels, and promote overall vitality.

While detoxing often involves dietary changes, supplements, and lifestyle modifications, self-assessment is a crucial aspect that is frequently overlooked.

Monitoring key indicators such as feces, urine, and body pH can provide valuable insights into the effectiveness of your detox regimen and your overall health status.

Self-assessment during a detox serves as a vital tool for gauging progress, identifying potential issues, and making informed adjustments to your regimen. Paying close attention to your body's signals and subtle changes, can optimize the detox process and ensure its safety and efficacy.

The appearance, color, and odor of feces and urine offer valuable clues about your digestive health, hydration status, and potential underlying issues.

Here's a breakdown of what to look for:

FECES COLOR CHART

- Brown: A healthy and normal color indicating efficient digestion.
- Green: May suggest rapid transit through the digestive tract or consumption of green foods.
- Yellow: Could indicate excess fat in the stool or issues with the liver or gallbladder.
- Black: Might signify bleeding in the upper digestive tract.
- Red: Could indicate bleeding in the lower digestive tract or consumption of red foods like beets.

URINE COLOR CHART

- Pale Yellow: Indicates good hydration and healthy kidney function.
- Dark Yellow: Signals mild dehydration and the need to increase fluid intake.
- Amber or Honey: Indicates severe dehydration and requires immediate rehydration.
- Cloudy: Could indicate a urinary tract infection or kidney stones.
- Red or Pink: May suggest blood in the urine, potentially indicating an infection or kidney issue.

Maintaining a balanced pH level in the body is essential for overall health and proper bodily function. Monitoring your body's pH level can provide insights into your acid-base balance and overall well-being.

BODY PH CHART

- Neutral pH (7.0): Indicates a balanced pH level.
- Acidic pH (Below 7.0): May indicate acidosis, caused by factors like diet or stress.
- Alkaline pH (Above 7.0): May indicate alkalosis, caused by factors like vomiting or certain medications.

Taking an integrated approach to health involves considering the interconnectedness of various bodily systems. It's important to discuss a range of diagnostic tests with your healthcare provider. By understanding your body's unique needs and addressing them through targeted diagnostics, you can work towards achieving optimal health and well-being.

Diagnostics and tests to ask for include:

COMPREHENSIVE BLOOD PANEL

- Complete blood count (CBC)
- Lipid profile (LDL, HDL, triglycerides)
- Blood glucose levels (fasting glucose and/or HbA1c)
- Liver function tests (AST, ALT, ALP, bilirubin)
- Kidney function tests (creatinine, BUN)
- Thyroid function tests (TSH, T3, T4)
- Vitamin and mineral levels (vitamin D, B12, iron, magnesium)

INFLAMMATORY MARKERS

- C-reactive protein (CRP)
- Erythrocyte sedimentation rate (ESR)
- Homocysteine levels

HORMONE LEVELS

- Testosterone (for both men and women)
- Estrogen (for women)
- Progesterone (for women)
- Follicle-stimulating hormone (FSH) and luteinizing hormone (LH)
- Cortisol levels (morning cortisol, cortisol rhythm)

NUTRITIONAL ASSESSMENT

- Micronutrient testing (vitamins, minerals, antioxidants)
- Omega-3 fatty acid levels
- Food sensitivity testing (IgG/IgE antibodies)
- Gut health assessment (stool analysis, digestive enzyme levels)

METABOLIC FUNCTION

- Metabolic panel (including markers for metabolic syndrome)
- Insulin sensitivity testing (e.g., fasting insulin, homeostatic model assessment for insulin resistance (HOMA-IR))
- Lipid particle size and density (advanced lipid testing)

CARDIOVASCULAR HEALTH

- Electrocardiogram (ECG/EKG)
- Stress testing (exercise stress test, stress echocardiography)
- Cardiac calcium scoring (for assessment of coronary artery calcification)

NEUROLOGICAL ASSESSMENT

- Neurotransmitter testing (serotonin, dopamine, GABA)
- Brain imaging (MRI, CT scan)
- Cognitive assessments (memory tests, cognitive function tests)

FUNCTIONAL MEDICINE ASSESSMENTS

- Comprehensive digestive stool analysis (CDSA)
- Adrenal function testing (salivary cortisol rhythm)
- Organic acids testing (for assessment of metabolic function and gut health)
- Heavy metal toxicity testing (urine or blood tests)

GENETIC TESTING

- DNA testing for assessing genetic predispositions to certain health conditions and personalized treatment approaches
- Pharmacogenetic testing to determine how your body metabolizes medications

LIFESTYLE ASSESSMENTS

- Sleep studies (polysomnography, home sleep apnea tests)
- Physical fitness assessments (cardiorespiratory fitness tests, body composition analysis)
- Stress assessment tools (questionnaires, heart rate variability analysis)

To effectively monitor your progress during a detox, consider incorporating regular self-assessment into your routine:

- Keep a Journal: Record daily observations of feces, urine, and body pH levels to track changes over time.
- Stay Hydrated: Maintain proper hydration to ensure accurate urine color and pH readings.
- Adjust Your Detox Plan: Use self-assessment results to modify your detox regimen as needed, such as adjusting dietary choices or supplement intake.
- Consult a Professional: If you notice significant changes or have concerns about your observations, seek guidance from a healthcare professional for personalized advice and support.

Self-assessment ensures effectiveness and safety of a detoxification journey. By paying attention to key indicators such as feces, urine, and body pH, you can gain valuable insights into your body's response to the detox process and take proactive steps to support your overall health and well-being.

CHAPTER 32: BECOME YOUR OWN HEALTH EXPERT

The first step in becoming your own health expert is to ensure you're fully stocked on everything you'll need to support your well-being.

By carefully selecting natural remedies, supplements, and healthcare products tailored to your needs, you empower yourself to take proactive steps toward self-care and holistic healing.

A well-equipped medicine cabinet serves as a foundation for your journey toward becoming more proactive, enabling you to address common ailments, support your body's natural healing processes, and cultivate overall vitality and resilience.

Here's what you should consider including in your holistic medicine cabinet:

- Colloidal Silver: Topical Use (10-20 PPM) - Effective for wound care and topical applications due to its antimicrobial properties. Internal Use (50-500 PPM) - Supports immune health and overall wellness when taken internally.

- Essential Oils: Various essential oils, such as

lavender, tea tree, peppermint, and eucalyptus, for aromatherapy, massage, and topical applications.

- Herbal Supplements: Natural supplements such as turmeric, ginger, echinacea, and elderberry for immune support, inflammation reduction, and overall health maintenance.

- Homeopathic Remedies: Homeopathic remedies for common ailments like Arnica for bruising and injuries, Oscillococcinum for flu symptoms, and Calendula for skin irritation.

- Tinctures and Herbal Extracts: Alcohol- or glycerin-based extracts of herbs, such as chamomile, valerian, and St. John's Wort, for various health concerns like stress, anxiety, and sleep disturbances.

- Probiotics with Prebiotics: Supplements containing a combination of beneficial bacteria strains (probiotics) and prebiotic fibers to support gut health, digestive function, and a balanced microbiome.

- Digestive Enzymes and Diatomaceous Earth: Digestive enzymes aid in the breakdown of food and support optimal digestion, while diatomaceous earth can help cleanse the digestive tract and support detoxification.

- Healing Salves and Balms: Natural topical remedies made from ingredients like beeswax, coconut oil, and herbal extracts for cuts, burns, insect bites, and skin irritations.

- Natural Pain Relief: Items like arnica gel, CBD oil, or white willow bark for pain relief and inflammation reduction.

- Healing Teas: Herbal teas like chamomile, ginger, peppermint, and green tea for relaxation, digestion, detoxification, and immune support.
- Natural First Aid Supplies: Bandages, gauze, adhesive tape, and antiseptic solutions like hydrogen peroxide or witch hazel for minor injuries and wound care.
- Mind-Body Wellness Tools: Meditation cushions, yoga mats, stress balls, or guided meditation CDs for promoting mental and emotional well-being.
- Books and Resources: Books on natural remedies, herbal medicine, holistic nutrition, and mindfulness practices for self-education and empowerment in holistic health care.
- Water Filtration Systems: Water filters or purifiers to ensure access to clean, contaminant-free water for drinking and cooking.

Always consult with a healthcare professional before starting any new supplements or treatments, especially if you have pre-existing health conditions or are pregnant/nursing.

△△△

In our quest for optimal health and well-being, we often find ourselves on a journey filled with twists and turns, challenges, and discoveries. As we navigate this path, we draw upon a wealth of resources, experiences, and insights to guide us towards greater vitality and resilience.

One invaluable resource on this journey is the knowledge

gained from firsthand experiences, particularly those related to detoxification. A good friend and colleague, Angela T. Moore, once told me, "I feel like it's our responsibility to share our own journeys."

It is, and I am. I encourage you to do the same.

Whether embarking on a structured detox program or adopting lifestyle changes to support the body's natural detoxification processes, these experiences offer valuable insights for you and others.

Tuning into our body's signals, honoring its innate wisdom, and making conscious choices, can support its natural ability to cleanse, rejuvenate, and heal.

Equally important is the guidance provided by healthcare practitioners who specialize in both allopathic and holistic approaches to health and wellness.

Part of being your own health expert is being your own health investigator and speaking to multiple experts to make the best decisions regarding your health.

Drawing upon a diverse array of modalities, including nutrition, herbal medicine, acupuncture, and mind-body practices, these practitioners offer a wealth of information that can be tailored to individual needs.

Foster a collaborative relationship with a trusted practitioner who listens, respects your journey, and empowers you. Together, you can navigate the complexities of modern healthcare with confidence and clarity.

△△△

In addition to professional guidance, the digital age has

ushered in a wealth of online resources and communities dedicated to health and wellness.

Online forums, social media groups, and hashtags on platforms like Twitter and TikTok provide opportunities to connect with others on similar health journeys, share experiences, and learn from collective wisdom.

By harnessing the power of these communities and tapping into shared knowledge, individuals can find support, inspiration, and encouragement along their path to wellness.

YouTube, with its vast array of health-related content, offers another avenue for learning and exploration. From informative videos on nutrition and exercise to guided meditations and yoga practices, YouTube provides a treasure trove of resources to support your health journey.

△△△

Offline, the support of family and friends plays a vital role in our health journey. By engaging in open and honest conversations about health struggles, sharing insights, and offering support, loved ones can become valuable allies in our quest for optimal well-being.

Exploring childhood health issues with parents and uncovering ancestral health insights can shed light on genetic predispositions, cultural influences, and familial patterns that impact our health today.

Furthermore, mastering the art of online research is essential for navigating the vast landscape of health information available on the internet.

By learning to discern credible sources from misinformation, leveraging informational websites, such as the CDC, NIH, and EWG, and seeking out evidence-based resources, individuals can empower themselves to make informed decisions about their health.

Seeking second and third opinions from healthcare professionals and exploring both holistic and allopathic treatment options can provide a well-rounded approach to healing and wellness.

△△△

Beyond these resources, health podcasts offer another valuable avenue for learning and exploration.

Platforms like Spotify, Apple Podcasts, Google Podcasts, and Stitcher host a wide range of health-focused podcasts covering topics such as nutrition, fitness, mental health, and holistic healing.

These podcasts offer insights from experts, inspiring stories of transformation, and practical tips for improving their health and well-being.

The journey to optimal health and well-being is multifaceted, dynamic, and deeply personal.

By integrating insights from all of these resources, you can navigate your own journey with confidence, resilience, and grace.

Everyone deserves that.

△△△

With my expertise in DNA swab analysis and virtual concierge coaching services, I aim to empower individuals to take control of their health and well-being.

I offer a range of DNA swab kits to cater to different health needs:

- The DNA general health kit offers comprehensive insights into overall health and wellness factors.
- The DNA drug report kit helps individuals understand how their genetics may influence their response to medications.
- The DNA estrogen kit focuses on genetic factors related to estrogen metabolism and hormonal balance.
- The DNA diet kit provides personalized dietary recommendations based on genetic predispositions.
- The DNA mind kit explores the genetic factors related to mental health and cognitive function.
- The DNA skin kit offers insights into genetic predispositions related to skin health and aging.
- The DNA sports performance kit provides information on genetic factors influencing athletic performance and recovery.

For more information, visit Detoxdayspa.com.

www.ingramcontent.com/pod-product-compliance
Lightning Source LLC
LaVergne TN
LVHW051726080426
835511LV00018B/2911